THE CANCER ECLIPSE

A Path of Hope Forward in Cancer Darkness

DAVID GRISSEN

Esophageal Cancer Survivor

Dave's Contact Information:

CancerEclipse@gmail.com
www.CancerEclipse.com

Unless otherwise indicated, Scripture quotations are from THE HOLY BIBLE, NEW INTERNATIONAL VERSION®, NIV® Copyright © 1973, 1978, 1984, 2011 by Biblica, Inc.® Used by permission. All rights reserved worldwide.

Scripture quotations marked (NLT) are taken from the Holy Bible, New Living Translation, copyright © 1996, 2004, 2007, 2013, 2015 by Tyndale House Foundation. Used by permission of Tyndale House Publishers, Inc., Carol Stream, Illinois 60188. All rights reserved.

Scripture quotations marked (NLV) are taken from the Holy Bible, New Life Version, copyright © Christian Literature International.

Scripture quotations marked (ISV) are taken from the Holy Bible: International Standard Version®. Copyright © 1996-forever by The ISV Foundation. ALL RIGHTS RESERVED INTERNATIONALLY. Used by permission.

Scripture quotations marked (ESV) are from the ESV® Bible (The Holy Bible, English Standard Version®), copyright © 2001 by Crossway, a publishing ministry of Good News Publishers. Used by permission. All rights reserved."

Scripture quotations marked (Berean Study Bible) are taken from The Holy Bible, Berean Study Bible, BSB, Copyright ©2016 by Bible Hub Used by Permission. All Rights Reserved Worldwide.

"Following a Chicken Leads to Healings in Indonesia" taken from: *Amazing Modern-Day Miracles*. Copyright © 2014 by Suzanne Frey. Published by Harvest House Publishers, Eugene, Oregon 97402. Used by Permission.

Cover Design by graphic artist, Steven Wold: stevenwold@yahoo.com.

Publishing help provided by Celeste Allen.

Thanks to both of you for the help!

Disclaimer: In this book I'm sharing my own medical story—how I went from cancer diagnosis to remission using medical, naturopathic, and spiritual means. In no way am I suggesting any type of medical or naturopathic treatment for you. Each of us is unique and must determine our own path forward. (DG)

Library of Congress Control Number: 1 2 3 8 910
Printed in the United States of America
ISBN-10: 1979612897
ISBN-13: 978-1979612890

To Sheri

You are the love of my life,
the greatest partner and caregiver to have in a
cancer eclipse!
We made it through this together!

To our wonderful Family

Your presence, support, and encouragement created the
desire to persevere!

.

CONTENTS

INTRODUCTION

I Hope You Don't Experience a "Cancer Eclipse!"

You head to the doctor because something's not right in your body. You have your examination and a barrage of tests. The further down the road they take you, the more anxiety and uncertainty overtakes you. And then finally— the results are in: It's the dreaded "C" word.

Your Life is Eclipsed by Cancer!

A few seconds after the doctor utters, "You have cancer," the "hope it isn't" is smashed. The joy recedes out of your life. The pit in your stomach grows. And the dreams and plans you made looking forward fall flat on the floor. You realize your life is making a major turn on the downhill slope of life.

It feels like you've entered a black hole where nothing is defined, nothing is certain. What lies ahead? Visions of saying goodbye to your spouse, family, and friends weigh down your spirit. It's like finding yourself in the dark center of an eclipse. Others might be seeing the sunshine, but you are numb, feeling nothing but despair and darkness.

That's the beginning of the cancer journey, and it's an ominous, negative place to be.

We live in Bend, Oregon—a town on the edge of the path of the August 22, 2017, total eclipse of the sun. So this past August, Sheri and I, along with two of our grandchildren, lined up our chairs outside on our lawn and through special glasses watched the moon slowly edge forward over the sun.

The brightness was slowly blocked, little by little, finally creating full darkness. It was an amazing sight that doesn't happen often.

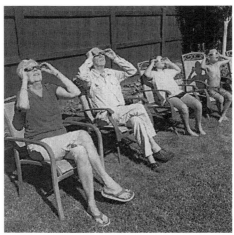

The sun is up there somewhere ...

As this eclipse developed before my eyes, I realized this is like my experience with cancer. In a "cancer eclipse" the darkness moves in step-by-step over your hope-filled, sunny life, creating an emotional, psychological, mental, spiritual, and practical "darkness."

After going through that initial shock of a cancer diagnosis, we do get our personal equilibrium back, so we can take on the coming battle against a strong enemy.

And we eventually realize that if the treatments we get can diminish or even end the cancer plague in our lives, we will see the sun re-emerge from the present darkness. We'll experience hope, joy, and expectation again!

We all know our lives are finite and temporary, but we don't think that way about them very often. At least, I never did. And we normally don't live with the mortal reality on our minds. Until the "C" word hits! Then the fact stated by a wise king takes hold: "Our days on earth are like grass; like wildflowers we bloom and die."[1]

The reality is, a cancer eclipse changes everything! We think about getting our house in order. Our kids start thinking about more time with us. The dreams with our spouse must be rearranged. In our minds, as we perceive the near-term future, life will absolutely not be the same.

My wife, Sheri, and I have both experienced "cancer eclipses." She's fought lymphoma cancer two times and has won the battle. In fact, a major victory for her was taking out her port after two years of clear scans. That port was the last vestige of a dark cancer eclipse. Now there was sunshine!

And I've just fought through my cancer battle with an esophageal tumor I finally had taken out. I'm on the victory side of that battle as well. My prognosis is good. The sun is out!

So I can testify, there can be life *with* cancer, life *without* cancer, and life *after* cancer. It's bleak when it hits. But through treatment—both medical and natural—we can still experience more time on this earth with the people we love before the grass is totally withered!

---

[1] King David, Psalm 103:15, The Holy Bible.

3

Unfortunately, esophageal cancer is on a slight increase today. The American Cancer Society's estimates for esophageal cancer cases in the United States for 2017 are:

- About 16,940 new esophageal cancer cases diagnosed (13,360 in men and 3,580 in women)

- About 15,690 deaths from esophageal cancer (12,720 in men and 2,970 in women)[2]

This disease is three to four times more common among men than among women. The lifetime risk of esophageal cancer in the United States is about 1 in 125 in men and about 1 in 435 in women. (See Chapter 2 for risk factors that can affect these statistics.)

Esophageal cancer makes up about 1% of all cancers diagnosed in the United States, but it's much more common in other parts of the world, such as Iran, North China, India, and South Africa.

The main type of esophageal cancer in those areas is squamous cell carcinoma. Squamous cell carcinoma develops in the flat cells that line the esophagus, typically in the middle or upper parts of the esophagus closer to the throat.

I ended up diagnosed with adenocarcinoma, the most common type of esophageal cancer in the USA. This type forms in glandular cells in the lining of the esophagus that release mucus close to the stomach. Mine was just above the hiatal valve.

---

[2] This stat takes into consideration all those who die because of esophageal cancer at some point in time, not only those who die in the same year.

Why I Wrote This Book

I specifically wrote this book for those 16,000 new cancer warriors who start their journey on this esophageal cancer road each year. But I'm sure it has application more broadly for other cancer patients as well, and especially for their caregivers, who want to be more informed on the path forward.

I believe each of us has our own unique cancer road to travel in our specific situation. After all, we're at different diagnostic stages. Our bodies are unique to us alone. We process the cancer eclipse differently based on our experience and personalities. We have different doctors and may get different advice based on their training and experience.

So, considering all these variables, my journey was and is unique to me. And your journey is unique to you. No one can make decisions for us or decide what's best for us. We each must discern and determine our journey forward ourselves.

This calls for wisdom on our part, not comparing our journey to others—which can either encourage us (I'm better off) or discourage us (I'm worse off), based on our opinion of their situation. If we have cancer, let's just admit it—we're in a bad situation and must devise our healing path forward in a way that makes sense to us!

At the same time, because we're all dealing with aberrant cancer cells, and they have been analyzed and treated by some very sharp people over decades, there are some medical protocols and principles in this journey which are the same for each of us. This brings hope to our bad situation.

The chemo types used have been tested on specific cells over time to ensure their demise.

The radiation used is more accurately delivered today because of better technology.

The operation to take out the tumor has been tested and become better developed over time. Even though it's a complex operation, it works. We just need a VERY competent doctor to do it. And our medical establishment has fostered the emergence of these VERY competent doctors!

In addition, in our specific cancer journeys, Sheri and I supplemented the medical (allopathic) with the natural (naturopathic).

We decided to use naturopathic medicine as well because the allopathic tends to focus on science and pharmaceuticals which can weaken the immune system. The naturopathic, on the other hand, focuses on nutrition that creates a strong immune system.

Our immune systems have kept us very healthy over our long lifespan. But now in our seventies, that body system has just about worn out. It has valiantly battled the toxins we've unwittingly or wittingly put into our mouths or lungs over all these years. If this system is not strengthened, it could be on its last legs.

The good news is we can bring our immune systems back out of weakness into some semblance of power.

Could there be enough immune power to overcome the cancer? That's a question for each of us to answer, and it tests our wisdom and knowledge. But foods and supplements do make a difference in this journey.

Since I was diagnosed with esophageal cancer in October 2014, and finally had the tumor taken out in March

2017, I've had the opportunity to talk with many others fighting this same cancer.

One of those is my friend, Tom, who had his operation before me. He and his wife Madeleine have been very helpful to Sheri and me as I struggled through the operation and recovery phases.

Others have contacted me after my operation to gain some insight and advice as they struggle through one phase or another.

Since I like to write, I decided to document my journey, decisions, wrestlings, questions, and cancer path, in this book, hoping to bring encouragement and some enlightenment to those of you still engaged deeply in this battle.

At least that's my desire—to be helpful to you—if you are in some phase of the cancer fight!

And my hope is that your cancer eclipse, while expressing darkness at a certain moment in time, will brighten up quickly into a longer life of hope and enjoyment for you!

1
SOMETHING I NEVER WANTED—A TUMOR!

I was moving forward positively at a good clip as I rolled into my seventh decade of life. Retirement was just around the corner.

At this time, Sheri and I were leading an organization, Life Impact, Inc. (www.LifeImpactMinistries.net). Several strategic trips were on our calendar. And we enjoyed time with our five children and their spouses and kids along the way. We could declare, "Life is good!"

My father lives in Inverness, Florida. So one of those trips in January 2014 was to visit him for his ninety-seventh birthday. On that travel docket, we put in another week on the Florida beaches to offset the cold, windy January winter we experience in Bend, Oregon.

The Cough That Never Quits!

I came back with a gentle cough which increased in intensity as we moved into February.

After a month of inability to stop it, and thinking I picked up some bug in Florida, I finally went to my general doctor. He prescribed an antibiotic to knock it out, which I took religiously. But the cough didn't go away. I was still plagued.

We tried a different antibiotic. This medicine should have knocked it out, but I kept gently coughing. This cough went on for eight months, with some relief during the summer.

But in the fall it came back again noticeably. At a social gathering one night in September, I explained to a doctor friend the persistent cough I could not defeat. Fortunately, he was an ear, eye, and nose specialist. He suggested it could be acid reflux irritating my throat.

What's a Barium Test?

Back to my general MD I went with this reflux suggestion. He thought it was a possibility and prescribed a barium test to see what the reality of reflux might be.

The technicians popped the liquid barium into my mouth while I was standing upright, pressed against an x-ray machine. The pictures were taken and analyzed...ouch...a tumor was spotted in the esophagus. Not good news!

So in my life, September 2014 was a good news month and a bad news month. The good news was the clear diagnosis of what caused my cough—glad to know that after ten months.

The bad news was the clear diagnosis of the tumor might be cancer—not sure I wanted to hear that! But the "C" fact still had to be verified. So on to the next diagnostic test I went.

My First Endoscopy

Immediately an appointment was set up for an endoscopy to determine the nature of the tumor. A few days later, into the local hospital I went again to have a snake pushed through my throat into my esophagus and stomach.

Fortunately, I went under anesthesia before the scope went down and some of the tissue was clipped. When I woke up the gastroenterologist confirmed the tumor as esophageal cancer!

A lab analysis followed the biopsy to further confirm what was I had been told. Soon we knew the type of cell the cancer was and its potential for growth. The "C" word was now my reality.

All the worst negative thoughts covered over the positive thoughts of my mind. How bad is this cancer? Will this take me to the grave? Do I only have a few months left with my wife and kids? What does this mean for the treatment going forward and the suffering I might have to go through?

I knew this would definitely change the basic trajectory of our life's plans.

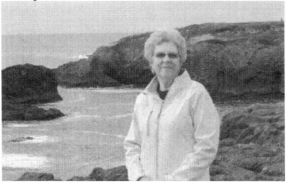

Sheri had fought through lymphoma cancer in late 2010 with chemo treatments for five months. I remembered how her energy was zapped and how much time she spent under a blanket by the fireplace, reading and sleeping. This was now my expectation for myself.

She did beat the cancer in early 2011, however, so some of my hope for the future returned as I thought of her unique battle with this crazy stuff.

My Second Endoscopy

At this time I was under the care of a local oncologist, Dr. William Martin. He set up an appointment in Portland, Oregon, for another endoscopy. I didn't realize before this how many variations there are on the endoscopic theme.

The endoscope was invented by a German doctor over 200 years ago; so it has a long history of development and use. I discovered the procedure is minimally invasive and quite safe in the hands of a competent doctor.

This second time my procedure was an ultrasound endoscopy. The purpose of this measurement was to determine the extent of the cancer and to "stage" it for me.

My Diagnosis

In his examination, the doctor first determined the tumor was "distal," or in the lower part of the esophagus. He also discovered the tumor had eaten through five of the seven layers of my esophagus and was close to breaking through into adjacent tissue—if it hadn't already.

To confirm possible metastasis[3] he noticed two lymph nodes adjacent to the outside layer of the esophagus were somehow infected.

Fortunately for me, while I was under anesthesia, a decision was made *not* to biopsy those two lymph nodes. This meant no needle had to be poked through the wall of the esophagus from the inside, potentially spreading the cancer through the procedure itself.

Two days later when I got these lab results back, I had to learn a new code language, the "staging" code, which in my case was, Stage II, T3 N1 MX.

The TNM Staging System

According to the National Cancer Institute,[4] the TNM system is the most widely used cancer staging system in the American medical establishment. Most hospitals and medical centers use it as their main method for cancer reporting. Exceptions to this are brain and spinal cord tumors and blood cancers.

If you are fighting cancer, you are probably well aware of your diagnosis and what it means. But I can't keep it straight so this info is included here for my future benefit as much as for yours!

In defining the TNM system, we see that…

---

[3] Metastasis is when a localized cancer breaks out of its original location into the blood supply, other adjacent tissue, or organs.

[4] Information from the National Cancer Institute, (https://www.nih.gov/about-nih/what-we-do/nih-almanac/national-cancer-institute-nci).

- *The T Factor* refers to the size and extent of the main tumor, which is usually called the primary tumor.

   Here is how the T factor is further defined:

   o TX = Main tumor cannot be measured.

   o T0 = Main tumor cannot be found.

   o T1, T2, T3, T4 = Refers to the size and/or extent of the main tumor. The higher the number after the T, the larger the tumor or the greater the extent it has grown into nearby tissues. Ts may be further divided to provide more detail, such as T3a and T3b. (In my case the tumor was large enough to be judged a size 3.)

- *The N Factor* refers to the number of nearby or "regional" lymph nodes identified with cancer.

   Here is how the N factor is further defined:

   o NX = Cancer in nearby lymph nodes cannot be measured.

   o N0 = There is no cancer in nearby lymph nodes.

   o N1, N2, N3 = Refers to the number and location of lymph nodes that contain cancer. The higher the number after the N, the more lymph nodes that contain cancer. (In my case the doc thought I had cancer in one lymph node without actually taking a biopsy of it. In my opinion it would have been more scientifically accurate to give me an NX versus an N1, but I'm sure they had good reasons for the N1. Err on the side of caution?)

- *The M Factor* refers to whether the cancer has metastasized, or spread from the primary tumor to other parts of the body. This is usually spotted through CT and PET scans.

The M factor may be further defined as:

- MX = Metastasis cannot be measured. (In my case, since no biopsy was done on the potentially cancerous lymph node, M1. The specialist didn't know if it had spread of not. Fortunately for me the CT and PET scans showed no metastasis. So again, in my opinion, MX would have been more scientifically accurate perhaps, except to err on the side of caution is best.)

- M0 = Cancer has not spread to other parts of the body.

- M1 = Cancer has spread to other parts of the body.

Another, less detailed, way to stage the cancer is to discuss it as a "Stage." There are five stages:

Stage 0 = Abnormal cells are present but have not spread to nearby tissue. This is also called carcinoma *in situ*, or CIS. This condition is not cancer but may become so.

Stage I, Stage II, and Stage III = Cancer is present. The higher the number, the larger the cancer tumor and the more it has spread into nearby tissues.

Stage IV = The cancer has metastasized or spread to distant parts of the body through adjacent tissue, the lymph system, or the blood system.

A Late Surprise for Me

So that's how the staging of cancer works and where I found myself with my specific staging numbers.

In my case, however, I was in for a big, personal, positive surprise two years later as I came out of the operation that took out my esophagus in a Seattle hospital.

The pathology of the tumor and seventeen lymph nodes, taken out and analyzed by a lab technician as the operation progressed, indicated my staging had actually gotten better. It went from the original Stage II, T3 N1 MX, to the actual reality of the tumor and lymph nodes, Stage I, T1 N0 M0.[5]

Why This Positive Change?

It is my opinion that this positive change occurred in my cancer situation because of some of the measures I took to fight the cancer during the period of time from diagnosis in September 2014 until my operation in March 2017.

(The only other option is that my original diagnosis was very much missing the mark!)

These elements of my fight create my unique story. No matter your diagnosis and staging, some of these measures might be very helpful to you as you travel your unique path against this disease. You decide as I share this.

---

[5] This staging number is based on the analysis and pathology of the operation. No gastroenterologist has changed the original staging because the operation made this irrelevant. An accurate staging number is still relevant for me, however, because I think about the changes in the tumor and what caused those. One reality has become another reality! Why?

2
MUST I GET DRUGGED & NUKED & CUT UP…REALLY?

I got used to going to the St. Charles Cancer Center in October 2010, when Sheri discovered a lymphoma tumor the size of a grapefruit in her neck. Before this we really enjoyed grapefruit!

Her oncologist's office was on the main floor of the Cancer Center, and the chemo infusion room was on the second floor. There were a few windows letting in light in a rather drab, sterile setting.[6]

Sheri spent much time there, and periodically I joined her. Often I found this experience a little unsettling, especially with all the patients hooked up to IV machines, sitting in lounge-type chairs, feet up with caps on their heads to cover bald skulls. And they had tired looks on their faces.

---

[6] Now the St. Charles Cancer Center is in a new building with a glassed-in infusion room, overlooking the beautiful Cascade Mountain range. It's a bright, cheery, and uplifting room. Sheri had her second set of chemo treatments there, and I had mine there also.

The cancer suffering was obvious—what a horrible disease—and yet with certain treatments, lives were extended and patients had more time with their families than they initially thought possible. Others, however, didn't make it.

Sheri is one of those who made it! Her chemo treatments took the fast-growing lymphoma down and out. Scans indicated cancer remission for five years. But on her fifth-year CT scan, a slower-growing lymphoma unfortunately showed up on the screen.

Back to the infusion room, this time the bright, cheery one. Additional treatments for this type of lymphoma cancer knocked it out as well. Her latest CT scan was clear, and she is doing great, in full remission.

So we've both been on the cancer trail, and this past time in 2015 we were doing it together! Our oncologist, Dr. William Martin, was tracking with both of us in what became our unique journey against cancer.

Dr. Martin, Tracking with Me

When my esophageal cancer was diagnosed, Dr. Martin was tracking with me each step of the way through the whole diagnostic process, offering encouragement, perspective, medical input, and setting up my specialist appointments. What a ton of appointments there were!

Once we knew the esophageal cancer was a reality in my body through the "scopes," we moved into his area of expertise—determining which treatment should be recommended to deal with my specific cancer.

This introduced me to the world of statistics attached to each treatment level I would encounter.

In my case, the normal cancer protocol was to first get chemo-radiation. Then six weeks after I finished those, I would head back into the hospital for a transhiatal esophagectomy.

In this operation, my esophagus, with the tumor in it, would be removed, and my stomach would be "re-sectioned" to form my new esophagus!

The World of Survival Statistics

In our consultations with Dr. Martin during Sheri's first lymphoma battle, we hit the mathematical world of cancer statistics. Cancer research has been tracking stats for years and computerizing the results. So medical professionals have access to many factors—one being survival rates.

In my research for this book I discovered an article by the American Cancer Society (ACS).[7] Fortunately, with improved treatments, survival rates are climbing. The stats below are from 2017, the year I'm writing this. I'm sure the ACS will continue to update this year-by-year; so google the URL in the footnote to get updated information.

Doctors often use survival rates as a standard way of discussing a person's prognosis (outlook). While giving a realistic view of this type of cancer, statistics are very objective and non-compassionate.

Personally, I don't like dealing with these numbers for any length of time because they can be depressing. And they are not an exact science anyway.

At the same time, you might be someone, like me, who gravitates toward information. I find that knowing where I

---

[7] ACS articles on various cancer statistics, (https://www.cancer.org/research/cancer-facts-statistics.html).

stand "centers" me on the inside and takes away doubts and anxiety.

Or perhaps you're a person who doesn't think the numbers would be helpful to you now.

So if you don't want to know the survival rates for esophageal cancer, please skip down to the next section "Statistics—Not an Exact Science."

Here Are the Unfortunate Esophageal Stats

Overall, the rates of esophageal cancer in the US have been fairly stable for many years with a slight uptick recently. The statistics show esophageal cancer was more common among African Americans than Caucasians, but now that has leveled off.

Squamous cell carcinoma is the most common type of esophageal cancer among African Americers, while adenocarcinoma is more common in Whites. Yet both types of esophageal cancer make up only 1% of all the cancer in the US diagnosed in a given year.

Each year in the USA there are about 16,940 new cases of both squamous and adenocarcinoma cancer diagnosed, of which over 13,360 are men and 3,580 are women.

The sad part of this is that 15,690 deaths also occur each year from this cancer—12,720 men and 2,970 women. The only silver lining to this statistic is that those passing away may have lived some years before their demise. That reality must be factored into the 15K number.

This does show the severity of this type of cancer, however. One attitude I noticed about myself when I was feeling good is that I probably didn't treat this with the seriousness it demanded. When I was feeling good, cancer was out of my mind. Feeling less than good created anxiety.

In my opinion, there's emotional space for hope and encouragement, even for Stage IV patients, when this type of personal protocol is followed:

1) both medical and natural treatments;
2) the multiplication of ongoing medical research which might produce a new treatment for me as time unfolds;
3) positive attitude;
4) anti-cancer diet;
5) exercise;
6) spiritual connection to God.

If you are reading this and don't have esophageal cancer, your lifetime risk factor of getting it is 1 in 125 if you're male (.008%), or 1 in 435 if you are female (.0068%). Not too much chance—**but be careful with ACID REFLUX!** *(The reasons are coming in these pages.)*

The American Cancer Society has listed fourteen risk factors that could affect you. Some are preventable, and others are fixed, like age.

Only 15% of those getting esophageal cancer are under the age of 55. See the footnote for the article about risk factors.[8]

How Long Might I Survive?

If you're fighting esophageal cancer today, the good news is, you're in for a better time than if you had it in the

---

[8] American Cancer Society article, "What are the Risk Factors for Cancer of the Esophagus?"
(https://www.cancer.org/cancer/esophagus-cancer/causes-risks-prevention/risk-factors.html).

1960s or 1970s. And progress on all fronts means those who follow us who have esophageal cancer now are in for a much better time fighting this than we are today.

In the 60s and 70s, only about 5% of patients survived at least five years after an esophageal diagnosis. Today that's up to an all-inclusive 20% who survive at least five years after diagnosis.

Caveat: This 20% number includes patients with all stages of the cancer. We do know that survival rate percentages are higher for those with early stage cancer and lower for later stage cancer. Therefore, in my opinion, it's more helpful to break out the stages and see survival rates attached to each stage. Again, this is not an exact science.

Another factor to consider in the survival rate is that researchers count all esophageal cancer patients within the past five-year period. Over that time period, many of these patients may have died of other causes besides their cancer and yet could be part of the statistic.

If that is the case, the actual overall survival rate of this cancer would be higher than 20%, which is good news.

Also, improvements in treatment since the time we were first diagnosed with cancer may result in a better survival rate for us going forward.

The unknown and scary issue for me is, which side of the statistic will I end up on—the 20% side or the 80% side? That's why anyone getting esophageal cancer should take this type very seriously and "number their days."

Discovering esophageal cancer in my body caused me to put my house in order and ensure that Sheri was able to function without me if I ended up in the 80% group and had only a short time to live.

Honing Down on the Statistics

To hone in on my specific statistic, it's more helpful to differentiate by stages rather than lumping all stages together into one statistic, as I said above.

Since I was Stage II, it is more helpful to know the survival rates for Stage II cancer, not just realize my general chances of making it to five years is 20%.

Unfortunately, survival rates are not readily available for each stage of the American Joint Committee on Cancer (AJCC) staging system for esophageal cancer.

What has been done, however, is to divide the statistics into three larger summary stages: (1) Localized, (2) Regional, and (3) Distant.

For this purpose, the National Cancer Institute (NCI) has created a database called SEER—Surveillance, Epidemiology,[9] and End Results. Statistics from SEER are based on patients diagnosed with esophageal cancer specifically between 2003-2009 and use the three categories mentioned above.

The stats below don't separate squamous cell cancer from adenocarcinoma (another inaccuracy factor), but those with the latter type are thought to have a slightly higher survival rate than listed below.[10] Here's how they shake out:

---

[9] Epidemiology is the branch of medicine that deals with the incidence, distribution, and possible control of diseases and other factors relating to health.

[10] ACS article, "Survival Rates of Cancer of the Esophagus by Stage", (https://www.cancer.org/cancer/esophagus-cancer/detection-diagnosis-staging/survival-rates.html).

Localized means the cancer is only growing in the esophagus. It includes AJCC Stage I and some Stage II tumors (T1, T2, or T3, N0, M0). Stage 0 cancers are not included in the statistics. The five-year survival rate for this group is 40%.

Regional means the cancer has spread to nearby lymph nodes or tissues. This includes T4 tumors and cancers with lymph-node spread (N1, N2, or N3). The five-year survival rate for this group is 21%.

Distant means the cancer has spread to organs or lymph nodes away from the tumor and adjacent lymph nodes, and includes all M1 (Stage IV) cancers. The survival rate for this group is 4%.

What If I Choose NOT to Do Part of the Full Protocol?

Since each of us has a unique path to walk in our specific life with cancer, there may be times we choose not to do one or more aspects of the medical cancer protocol. In my case I chose against the esophagectomy for two years for personal reasons I'll explain as we go along.

Here are some options in regard to the normal esophageal cancer protocol:

Radiation alone. This option is most often chosen when a patient cannot have surgery for some reason. The one-year survival rate for doing only radiation to nail the tumor is 18%. After two years the survival rate for this option is 8%.

When radiation is used as a way to control symptoms of esophageal cancer in stages III or IV it is a very effective. Seventy percent of these patients will experience a decrease in painful swallowing and other symptoms after radiation therapy.[11]

At the same time, if we *combine radiation with chemotherapy*, survival rates improve. For example, stage III esophageal cancer patients treated with both chemotherapy and radiation therapy have a 20% to 30% survival rate at three years rather than 18% at one year, or 8% at two.

[Note: As you will see from this book, for a couple reasons I decided not to do the surgery after chemo-radiation. Statistically, that decision dropped my survival rate from 40% to 30%.]

Statistics—Not an Exact Science

While these statistics can create a modicum of fear in any of us, we must remember they are not an exact science. These figures are the best the medical researchers can do through their tracking and the best facts they can use to create a realistic picture of what a patient faces.

One reason statistics aren't an exact science is because there are so many other factors to each person's unique cancer situation that are not, or cannot be, measured.

We can say with accuracy that adenocarcinoma tumors are located in the distal esophagus near the stomach.

Yet their size, type of cell, extent of penetration through the wall of the esophagus, infection of adjacent lymph nodes, effectiveness of the treatment, general health

---

[11] "Treating Esophageal Cancer with Radiation Therapy" by Diane Rodriguez, from *Everyday Health*,
(http://www.everydayhealth.com/esophageal-cancer/radiation-therapy-for-esophageal-cancer.aspx).

condition of the patient, and DNA all play an important part in our specific cancer journeys.

Most of these factors are not taken into consideration in determining survival rates.

Also in the mix is the decision of our oncologist to use a certain type of chemo. While there is "best practice" indicating which type of chemo should be given in a specific situation, this is still a subjective call on our oncologist's part.

And at any given time in the dynamic medical research realm, new chemo types and other products are being developed to challenge present best practice.

I can imagine a competent oncologist must spend much time today reading clinical trial results and other reports in order to stay current in this accelerated research field. Only then can wise direction be given to their patients and solid decisions made about treatment.

An Example of the Dynamic Research Environment Today

Recently I read an email sent from the Leukemia and Lymphoma Foundation. This foundation was helpful to us in 2010 by providing grant money to offset some of the costs of Sheri's first lymphoma battle.[12]

Here's an example, from their email, of what I just mentioned about accelerated cancer research:

---

[12] If you face rising bills for cancer treatments, check with the financial office of your cancer treatment center for this type of grant. There is probably money or discounted treatment options to help you get through this valley financially. In our case, Medicare covered the total amount after we reached age 65.

Advanced cancer research can take many twists and turns, and sometimes an approach that's been discounted by others proves to be surprisingly fruitful.

In 2009, John C. Byrd, MD, of The Ohio State University started to research the effectiveness of a drug, ibrutinib, on chronic lymphocytic leukemia (CLL). While many experts predicted his approach would not be effective, clinical trials showed unprecedented response rates to this drug.

As a result, ibrutinib was approved for patients with relapsed or refractory CLL in 2014. But the story continues! A study last year by an LLS Specialized Center of Research (SCOR) team, led by Tom Kipps, MD, UCSD, resulted in FDA approval of ibrutinib as a front-line treatment for CLL patients.[13]

If I were an oncologist today (instead of an oncologist wannabe), I would have to be aware of these types of developments in the field, or my way of treating this disease would not be as effective for the patient as it should.

Another factor that cannot be measured and put into the survival rates are the sneaky ways of cancer itself.

These unorthodox cell masses don't show up on CT or PET scans unless they're a certain size.[14] So they could be

---

[13] Leukemia & Lymphoma Society email article to supporters, May 16, 2017, (http://www.lls.org).

[14] This and more info from ACS webpage "Imaging (Radiology) Tests for Cancer.": "Tumor size imaging tests can often be very helpful, but they have limits. For instance, most of the time, these tests alone can't show for sure if a change is caused by cancer. Imaging tests can find large groups of cancer cells, but no imaging

lurking in the body planning no good for us without being detected. This reality causes oncologists to use the word "remission" rather than the word "cure."

You probably have other unique factors as well as these.

One of the unique factors in my case was my wait time to have the operation. My surgeon, Dr. Brant Oelschlager, had two months of operations booked. Waiting two months opened me to the possibility of metastasis.

Therefore, Dr. Oelschlager, wanted me to have several chemo treatments in the meantime to ensure the cancer would not metastasize while I was waiting.

In 2014 after my diagnosis, I had Cisplatin chemo with the radiation treatments. Because of these stresses on my cancer cells and their fight for life, they morphed from their original form into a HER-2 cell that is similar to a common type of breast cancer cells. For HER-2 a chemo called Herceptin is very effective.

So Dr. Martin had that chemo infused into my veins every third week in my waiting period.

The Herceptin was enhanced with a second chemo, Xeloda. I had to take six Xeloda pills a day for twelve days after each Herceptin treatment.

These issues—the waiting period plus additional two chemos for a certain period of time—were not factored into the survival rates but could certainly have affected my outcome up or down.

---

test can show a single cancer cell or even a few. In fact, it takes millions of cells to make a tumor big enough to show up on an imaging test."
(https://www.cancer.org/treatment/understanding-your-diagnosis/tests/imaging-radiology-tests-for-cancer.html).

Principle Learned About Medical Treatment

I also learned an important principle in this journey: It was wise for me to take charge of my own treatment by doing research, asking questions, and gently challenging medical suggestions with both data and personal uncertainties.

Whereas many doctors would be threatened by this patient approach, my oncologist, Dr. William Martin, is a very emotionally secure doctor who welcomed these questions from me.

Most often I would go with his opinions, but there were times when I didn't have inner peace about a prescribed path and, thus, raised my concerns.

He took my thoughts and questions seriously and worked with me to make appropriate changes. And although he couldn't recommend natural treatments to us because of the lack of scientific studies to verify outcomes, he was curious and encouraging when we decided to take time out from the medical track for those treatment options.

At one point I asked him, "I've been challenging you on a lot of issues along the way, will you continue to be my doctor even if I still push off the operation again and do a natural treatment in Mexico?" His answer was an enthusiastic, "Yes, because I'm YOUR doctor."

While we were in Mexico for twenty days of natural treatments at the CIPAG Clinic with Dr. Castillo, I met many other patients there as well. I heard several horror stories of how their oncologists would berate them and even cut off treatment if they decided to try some natural option or raised questions about some medical opinion.

How do we, as common patients, understand and relate to this type of attitude on the part of a professional? This is hard to understand. It would seem they are either very arrogant or very insecure.

My suggestion is if a doctor can't handle some gentle pushback and must have the dogmatic answer to every medical issue and opinion without question, you should probably find another doctor. Why put up with that attitude? It could actually be counter-productive and cause you harm!

Doctors are not infallible beings. They can make mistakes. So take charge of your life. Working together, in harmony with our doctor on our unique cancer reality is the best path forward—emphasis on "together" and "in harmony."

To have an understanding and secure doctor is a medical blessing! May their tribe increase!

Second Guessing the Protocol

As my treatment options became clear, the statistics were a major factor in the decisions about my future path. A 20% or 30% or even 40% survival rate was not too encouraging for my longevity.

And I simply couldn't envision myself without an esophagus. Nor could I wrap my mind around the reality of having my chest chewed up. We weren't created that way, I thought, so this can't be the right path for me to go.

How much basic fear of becoming disabled in some way or the fear of not making it through the operation factored into my thinking, I'm not sure. (Nine percent of those having the esophagectomy die within thirty days of the operation.)

Dr. Martin was clear on one fact: If I didn't follow the protocol there was no way medically to overcome the cancer. Then I would be limited to only palliative care instead of a possible cure.

So following his advice, I went to visit with Dr. Linyee Chang, the lead radiologist at the St. Charles Cancer Center in Bend, Oregon.

I would need radiation before the operation anyway, so I could push off for a short time that horrendous decision. But I would have to make it eventually. If it was a "yes" decision, my stomach would then become my new esophagus.

3

OKAY...HERE COMES THE NUCLEAR OPTION!

By the time I had my first appointment with Dr. Chang, I did some internet searching to check out the types of radiation I could have. You can find this info on the web yourself via Google, but for the sake of saving you time, and documenting this for me, I'm giving it to you here. This information comes from the National Cancer Institute[15] and the American Cancer Society.[16]

Most esophageal cancer treatments are of the (1) *external beam radiation therapy* variety. This was my stereotype of radiation—the external machine that turns and whines and NAILS YOU internally with a nuclear beam—and hopefully in the right location!

---

[15] NCI website:
(https://www.cancer.gov/about-cancer/treatment/types/radiation-therapy).

[16] ACS website:
(https://www.cancer.org/treatment/treatments-and-side-effects/treatment-types/radiation/basics.html).

Other types of radiation treatments I discovered were

(2) *internal beam or brachytherapy*, where radioactive material is PLACED IN the body near cancer cells, and

(3) *systemic radiation therapy* using radioactive substances like radioactive iodine which TRAVELS IN the blood to kill cancer cells.

The statistic regarding radiation is that over half of the cancer patients under doctor's care receive some form of radiation. That's 60% of us getting nuked at some point in our cancer treatment.

I knew St. Charles Cancer Center had these external radiation machines, so I thought this would be the type of treatment I would have. What I didn't realize until my research is there are a number of types of external beam radiation therapy. Only a consultation with Dr. Chang would clarify her recommendation for me.

PHoton Beam Therapy — The Standard External Beam Therapy

External-beam radiation therapy is most often delivered in the form of photon beams (either gamma rays or x-rays). A photon is the basic unit of light and other forms of electromagnetic radiation. It can be thought of as a bundle of energy.

The amount of energy in a photon bundle can vary. For example, the photons in gamma rays have the highest energy, followed by the photons in x-rays.

X-rays are the type of energy used most often in conventional radiation therapy. The electromagnetic waves in x-rays pass through most objects because of their physical properties.

But this type of radiation can also damage healthy tissue in the body. So doctors often reduce x-ray doses from the optimal cancer-fighting level to protect surrounding healthy tissue from harm.

Radiation machines have developed over the years to produce two ways to deliver external beam therapy. The machines delivering photon therapy are called, "linear accelerators". There are two types of these machines.

Intensity-Modulated Radiation Therapy (IMRT)
IMRT targets tumors more accurately than conventional radiation therapy. Using computers and 3-D images from CT scans, doctors focus small radiation beams on and around the tumor. This is a highly targeted treatment so that surrounding organs aren't affected.

Image-Guided Radiation Therapy (IGRT)
IGRT molds radiation beams to the contours of your tumor. Doctors use CT scans, ultrasound, or other guidance systems during each treatment to deliver more precise doses. This helps to ensure that the natural movement of the esophagus doesn't affect the treatment.

PRoton Beam Therapy—More Radiation with Less Risk

Another type of radiation therapy comes from protons (as opposed to photons). The proton is a positively charged atomic particle. These particles are raised to a high level of energy by a machine called a "particle accelerator." At this high energy level these protons are capable of destroying cancer cells.

An advantage of this type of therapy is that it can be much more accurately targeted to the cancer tumor without a lot of scarring of surrounding tissue. Unlike the photons in x-rays, proton beams stop after releasing their energy within their target.

A proton beam can be much more finely controlled, so higher doses of radiation can be safely delivered to tumors with less risk to healthy tissue.

Proton therapy is often the preferred option for treating solid tumors in children because protons can be controlled precisely. That means there is less radiation of normal tissues, helping prevent serious complications and lessening the chance of secondary tumors.

Besides effectiveness for children, studies show proton therapy to be effective in treating many types of tumors, including tumors of the prostate, brain, head, and neck, base-of-skull tumors, tumors near the spine, central nervous system, lung, gastrointestinal system, melanoma of the eye, as well as cancers that cannot be removed completely by surgery.

In addition to cancer treatment, proton therapy has been effectively used to treat Parkinson's disease, epilepsy, macular degeneration, arteriovenous malformations, several rheumatologic conditions and seizure disorders.[17]

Proton therapy has not yet been compared with standard external-beam radiation therapy in clinical trials. In addition, because the proton radiation machines are so expensive, many smaller treatment centers, like our center at St. Charles, do not offer proton treatment.

---

[17] *Proton Therapy Today,* (http://www.proton-therapy-today.com).

Neutron Therapy

Neutron therapy is a highly effective form of radiation therapy. Long-term experience with treating cancer has shown that certain tumor types are very difficult to kill using conventional radiation therapy. Those tough tumors are classified as being "radio-resistant."

Neutron therapy specializes in treating inoperable, radio-resistant tumors occurring anywhere in the body.[18]

In general, radiation therapy uses penetrating beams of ionizing radiation, primarily to treat cancerous/malignant tumors. The basic effect of ionizing radiation is to destroy the ability of cells to divide by damaging their DNA strands.

For photon and proton radiation treatments, the damage is done primarily by activated radicals produced from atomic interactions. This type of radiation is called *low Linear-Energy-Transfer* radiation (low LET).

Neutrons, however, are *high Linear-Energy-Transfer* radiation (high LET), and the damage is done primarily by the nuclear interactions themselves. If a tumor cell is damaged by low LET radiation, it has a good chance to repair itself and continue to grow. With high LET radiation, the chance for a damaged tumor cell to repair itself is very small.

---

[18] Neutron therapy is hard to find. "UW Medical Center is one of three facilities in the United States to offer neutron therapy, an especially powerful kind of radiation therapy shown to be effective against salivary gland tumors and some other forms of cancer."
(https://www.seattlecca.org/diseases/salivary-gland-cancer/treatment-options/neutron-therapy).

In general, fast neutrons can control very large tumors, because unlike low LET radiation, neutrons do not depend on the presence of oxygen to kill the cancer cells.

In addition, the biological effectiveness of neutrons is not affected by the time or stage in the life cycle of cancer cells, as it is with low LET radiation.

It often happens that large tumors have metastasized (spread) to other parts of the body before the patient seeks treatment. In these cases, neutrons can be used to control the primary tumor, but chemotherapy must be used to limit the spread of cancer through the rest of the body.

This treatment has been found particularly effective on cancers in the head and neck: for example, salivary glands, tongue, pharynx, oral cavity, and the nasopharynx. Neutron treatment in the chest is for mediastinum, pleura, and lungs.

In the abdomen and pelvis, neutron radiation therapy is effective against prostate, kidney, or uterine cancer. It can handle melanoma tumors, and if needed, works for "palliative care" of large, incurable tumors and metastasis from neutron-sensitive tumors.

Because the biological effectiveness of neutrons is so high, the required tumor dose to kill cancer cells is about one-third the dose required with photons or protons. A full course of neutron therapy is delivered in only 10 to 12 treatments, compared to 25-40 treatments needed for low LET radiation.

From this description, it appears esophageal cancer is normally not treated with neutron radiation. However, perhaps it could be put on the table for discussion with your radiologist to hear the rationale for not using it.[19]

---

[19] Fermi National Accelerator Laboratory (part of the American Physical Society) website,

Also, friends you may know with other types of cancers could be made aware of this option to discuss with their radiologist.

Wow! Our Medical System is Amazing— Other Radiation Treatments

According to the National Cancer Institute there are a number of other types of radiation treatments besides the three already mentioned:[20]

Tomotherapy: This is a type of image-guided IMRT. A tomotherapy machine is a hybrid between a CT imaging scanner and an external-beam radiation therapy machine. The part of the tomotherapy machine that delivers radiation for both imaging and treatment can rotate completely around the patient in the same manner as a normal CT scanner.

Stereotactic Radiosurgery: Stereotactic radiosurgery (SRS) can deliver one or more high doses of radiation to a small tumor. SRS uses extremely accurate image-guided tumor targeting and patient positioning. Therefore, a high dose of radiation can be given without excess damage to normal tissue.

However, SRS can be used to treat only small tumors with well-defined edges. It is most commonly used in the

---

(https://www.aps.org/programs/outreach/history/historicsites/fermilab.cfm).

[20] This information from the NCI article, "Radiation Therapy for Cancer, (https://www.cancer.gov/about-cancer/treatment/types/radiation-therapy).

treatment of brain or spinal tumors and brain metastases from other cancer types. For the treatment of some brain metastases, patients may receive radiation therapy to the entire brain (called whole-brain radiation therapy) in addition to SRS.

Stereotactic Body Radiation Therapy: Stereotactic body radiation therapy (SBRT) delivers radiation therapy in fewer sessions, using smaller radiation fields and higher doses than 3D-CRT, in most cases.

By definition, SBRT treats tumors that lie outside the brain and spinal cord. Because these tumors are more likely to move with the normal motion of the body, and therefore, cannot be targeted as accurately as tumors within the brain or spine, SBRT is usually given in more than one dose. SBRT can be used to treat only small, isolated tumors, including cancers in the lung and liver.

Electron beams are used to irradiate superficial tumors, such as skin cancer or tumors near the surface of the body, but they cannot travel very far through tissue. Therefore, they cannot treat tumors deep within the body.

My Personal Radiation Track

My visit with Dr. Chang went well as we discussed options and some of my questions regarding various types of radiation. St. Charles Cancer Center does not have a proton radiation machine. If I had chosen that option, I would have had to go to some other center and city for treatment.

Dr. Chang convinced me, however, that in my case it would be better to have a little "radiation scatter" rather than a very targeted, concise beam. The reason was because some cancer cells might be growing in the areas around the specific tumor site and would then possibly be nailed by this "scatter." That made sense to me, so I chose to do that.

Jumping into the Nuclear Fray

Once the decision had been made to move forward with this type of radiation (photon, IMRT), the next step was to simulate the radiation treatments I would soon be getting.

The skilled technicians first crafted my personal foam "body saddle". This tool made sure I was comfortable and had my body lying in exactly the same way every time I went on the table. This was one factor to ensure accuracy of the radiation treatment.

It was important to me to ensure my name was on MY saddle. And I made sure the technicians knew my name well. I didn't want them to inadvertently give me John Doe's saddle at some point! He might need brain radiation and I didn't want any of my brain fried. My family says I can't afford to lose any more of it anyway!

Because my past scans showed the exact location of the tumor in my chest, the technician could put a permanent "black dot" on my chest at the center of the tumor. This dot lined up the radiation machine accurately each time.

That ensured the same pattern of radiation would be delivered to the same points of the tumor and my chest in each of the following treatments.

Once this procedure had been completed, Dr. Chang and her team went to work to prepare the computer path. Then they determined the number of treatments I needed and amount of radiation I should have each time. In my case it was twenty-six treatments.

Prior to my first treatment, Dr. Chang consulted with me and shared more specifics and even the computer simulation of my radiation. I was now finally ready to get nuked!

Hooked Up to a Chemo Machine, Too?

As we know, however, the medical protocol for esophageal cancer was not just radiation, but chemo and radiation.

Dr. Martin informed me recent medical trials showed chemo infusion treatments along with the radiation protocol sensitized the cancer cells to better absorb the radiation. Having both, therefore, would improve survival rates over just radiation.

Of course, I then had another decision to make. Do I accept this recommendation by adding a two-hour chemo infusion each week prior to my series of radiation treatments?

I had not experienced chemo myself up to that point but saw the tremendous wear and tear of chemo on Sheri's body five years before. Did I want to put myself into this position? How would my body tolerate it—it was a chemical, after all.

I discovered the conclusion of the studies was quite strong:

> Concurrent therapy with the chemos—cisplatin and fluorouracil—along with radiation is superior to radiation therapy alone in patients with localized carcinoma of the esophagus. This was measured by control of local tumors, distant metastases, and

survival, but also came at the cost of increased side effects.[21]

Since my goal in taking treatment in the first place was to hopefully spend a few more years on this earth with Sheri, my family, and friends, I decided to take the chemo treatments and enhance the radiation. It was not a difficult decision from any angle.

So on the day my radiation treatments started, I traipsed up the stairs of the St. Charles Cancer Center to the infusion room, grabbed a chair with the mountain vista in view, got the needle in my vein (yes, I didn't need a port or pic line), and went to sleep for a couple hours while the chemo slowly flowed into my body.

Fortunately, the chemo was mild and my body tolerated it well with no side-effects for the six treatments I had.

Twenty-Six Times on the Table!

After receiving the chemo, I walked back down the stairs and over to the radiology department to start my radiation treatments. Pleasant staff greeted me. I had to give them my name and birthdate to ensure their computer program was correct for me. Very glad to do that!

---

[21] These results from "Medline ® Abstracts for References 36-38," 'radiation therapy, chemo-radiotherapy, neo-adjuvant approaches, and postoperative adjuvant therapy for localized cancers of the esophagus.' Wolters Kluwer, (http://www.uptodate.com/contents/radiation-therapy-chemoradiotherapy-neoadjuvant-approaches-and-postoperative-adjuvant-therapy-for-localized-cancers-of-the-esophagus/abstract/36-38).

Classical music was chosen to waft through the room and keep me peaceful. And I was ushered in and placed on my saddle.

Ash, my radiologist, left my room and soon the radiation machine clicked into gear. Quietly whining around me, it clicked, started, stopped, and started again. This process continued for 15 minutes. Often I would doze off as I relaxed, or think about some issue facing me that day, or simply pray quietly.

These radiation visits continued from early November 2014, until January 6, 2015. I hit a couple holidays during that time, so some weeks my regimen was four treatments instead of five. Needless to say, I was glad to be ending as 2015 started!

Watch Out for the Side Effects of Radiation!

In one of my early consultations about radiation with Dr. Chang, I was informed of the potential side effects of the targeted radiation. This introduced me to the reality that sometimes in allopathic medicine, the cure is worse than the illness, or the bark is worse than the bite.

I was informed that some of these side effects occur during the treatment and others might show up later in life.

Scar tissue interfering with body functions could be one of those.

In my case one acute effect I was warned about was *skin irritation* at the site of the treatment. This could show up as a red burn or dry and itchy skin. If this occurred, I was to treat it with a special salve they gave me in small tubes.

Fatigue is another common side effect of radiation therapy, regardless of which part of the body is treated. So I expected to take daily naps each day along with those nuke sessions. I figured a 15-30 minute walk each day would also be another anti-fatigue measure.

Sometimes *nausea* also sets in but usually with lower abdomen radiation. I did have some anti-nausea medicine however, because I was also getting the chemo that can cause the same effect.

I was also warned to watch out for *dehydration*. Drinking plenty of water as I went through this treatment was recommended.

Finally, the side effect I feared the most, was the *burn* inside my esophagus, making it difficult to swallow food because of the pain. Dr. Chang informed me that after about ten treatments I would start to feel a burn in the throat when I ate. For this I had a liquid to deaden the throat from pain.

Then Dr. Chang informed me that going further in the treatment regimen would mean enough burning so I ultimately might not be able to get any food down the esophagus. In this case a nose tube would be inserted into the stomach through my nostril so nutrition could be pushed into my body to keep me alive.

As you can imagine, I was not very happy picturing myself walking around with a tube hanging out of my nose. That's just what other people want to see…NOT.

However, this gave me the visual picture of sitting at home in my comfortable chair with a stack of books, reading my day away, and pushing liquid food down through my nose. Fortunately, we were moving toward Christmas time. So the house would be cozy with our fireplace on!

In What Condition Did I Come Through the Radiation?

As I got on the radiation table for the first time and into my saddle, I discovered this treatment was a piece of cake. No strain. No pain. Much gain. Good conversation with the technicians. Great music. In and out in 15 minutes!

As the number of treatments ticked off, I was waiting for the side effects to kick in. I was probably a little more tired than normal, but the BIG worry for me was still the eating issue.

The night before I started the regimen of twenty-six nuke arrows, Sheri and I went out for a steak dinner. I was afraid a T-bone would be out of my diet in the very near future.

Two weeks and ten treatments came and went. I was still eating everything I wanted.

Thanksgiving was coming up, so my family decided to celebrate it a week early for my eating benefit. We were all hoping I could enjoy turkey and the pumpkin pie. At that time, I was still eating everything offered me without esophageal pain, so I enjoyed the early celebration.

Then the actual Thanksgiving holiday arrived. Hey, I was still eating everything with no burning in my throat or esophagus. So in 2014, I actually celebrated Thanksgiving two times! An extra turkey had to bite the dust for me! Sorry, Mr. Turkey!

The next issue was Christmas. I thought, surely I would not be eating by the 25th of December. So again, my family, in deference to me and my appetite, set our Christmas celebration early. The date was the 18th of December, and the hope was I could still eat a little with my mouth at that time. Christmas ham surely tastes better through the mouth than a nose tube!

On December 18 we packed up and headed on our three-hour drive across the mountains from Bend to Oregon City, Oregon, where two of my daughters live.

We had a wonderful time together, and guess what? I was still not experiencing the burn syndrome and ate anything I wanted at our early Christmas party—including the great desserts! Wow!

Then the actual Christmas Day arrived on December 25. I was still eating everything with no burning anywhere in my esophageal tract.

So in 2014, I actually celebrated Christmas two times! Over this Christmas holiday, the food sacrifice on my behalf was either, two hogs offering a leg or one hog offering both legs. Sorry for them! Happy for me!

But I still had seven more radiation treatments to go to be finished on January 6, 2015. Since I wasn't finished yet, there was still the chance the burning would start. I kept my fingers crossed and kept praying against that.

On January 6, I entered the Cancer Center for my last radiation treatment. I was jubilant as were the technicians. *I had come through the twenty-six treatments without ANY side effects except a little fatigue!*

Ash told me in twenty-two years of working in the radiology department, I was only the second person he'd seen come through the treatments in such great shape.

I definitely remember January 6 was my last radiation treatment because that date happens to be my birthday. To celebrate, Sheri and I got into the car, after saying "thank you" and "good-bye" to the technicians with a couple dozen donuts, and headed out to a restaurant for...you guessed it…a steak dinner! Steak started my radiation journey and steak actually ended that journey!

Why Do I Think I Skated Through the Radiation?

To what do I attribute my very successful path through chemo-radiation? Since I know how I processed my radiation time and what my thoughts were, I must give the credit of my incredible radiation journey to God's hand of protection and healing on my body.

I am a follower of Jesus, the Messiah, and have been since I was nineteen years old. As soon as the cancer diagnosis hit me, I was actively seeking His healing hand on my life, all through my cancer journey, and continue that even now, post-operation.

It is my view that my radiation success is one example of His healing reality in my life over the past three years.

I don't know what your spiritual orientation or commitments are, so you may not be interested in how the spiritual intersected with the medical in my case. But it actually is the centerpiece and foundation of what I've experienced.

However, in order to respect your spiritual viewpoint whatever that might be, I'm not saying much about the spiritual impact on my cancer eclipse in the first eight chapters of this book. I want to ensure you see clearly how I managed the practical side of my cancer eclipse. The first eight chapters cover that in some detail.

If you are interested in seeing how I believe God was with me and helped me through all of this, I have documented the spiritual aspects of my journey in the final

Chapters (9-12) of this book, with a little more information in four of the Appendices (C, D, E, and F).

What's the Path Ahead?

As I got off the radiation table after my final treatment on January 6, 2015, I knew I still faced another ominous decision—should I have the horrendous esophagectomy operation or not? Emotionally I still could not envision what that step would mean for my life.

Because I had followed a very strong spiritual path during my cancer experience to this point, I thought perhaps I had been supernaturally, instantaneously healed from cancer by a spiritual touch of "Jehovah Rapha's" hand.[22]

My objective evidence for this view of healing was how I skated through the radiation without side effects, as I just documented. That gave me pause to think something supernatural had happened.

This spiritual inclination that I might be already healed of the cancer in a supernatural way led both Sheri and me to the idea that perhaps natural treatments could now control any cancer cells that might still be there, if there were any. This led us down another interesting path of life and treatments as we dealt with this crazy cancer eclipse.

---

[22] *Jehovah Rapha* is one of the Old Testament names for Yahweh, God of the Israelites, found in Exodus 15:26, "He said, 'If you listen carefully to the LORD your God and do what is right in his eyes, if you pay attention to his commands and keep all his decrees, I will not bring on you any of the diseases I brought on the Egyptians, for I am the LORD, who heals you.'" Cf: Jeremiah 3:22; 31:17; Isaiah 30:26; 61:1; and Psalm 103:3.

4
TO OPERATE OR NOT TO OPERATE?
THAT IS THE QUESTION!

We found the University of Washington Hospital Parking Garage, pulled in, got out, hit the door lock, and headed for the elevator.

Our objective: Dr. Brant Oelschlager's office on the fourth floor of the University Hospital. We checked in and waited for our appointment time.

Dr. Oelschlager is an Esophageal Surgeon and also a Professor of Surgery, specializing in esophagectomies for the past twenty years since he started his practice.

In fact, he has helped pioneer simplifying techniques of esophagectomy surgery, using laparoscopic methods to loosen the stomach and esophagus from their blood vessels.

This allows for a shorter operation time, which is less invasive, eliminating much trauma to the body. It also eliminates the chest drainage tubes of other approaches, which are highly invasive. The end result is quicker healing times and faster release from the hospital.

In addition, Dr. Oelschlager and several colleagues realized that post-operative care was very critical in survival rates. The national average of patients who die within thirty days of the operation is 9%.

Therefore, to lower that average for themselves, they spent time developing a care plan based on progress indicators for each day a recovering patient spends in the hospital. This lowered their average to 1%.

All of their after-care personnel are trained in moving this healing path forward. In addition, the interns, who make daily rounds to esophageal patients, are trained to evaluate healing success based on these factors.[23]

Dr. Oelschlager used the minimally invasive transhiatal esophagectomy method for my operation very effectively.

In the transhiatal esophagectomy, the esophageal tumor is removed through abdominal incision, without thoracotomy (going into the chest), and a left neck incision. The esophagogastric anastomosis (new stomach-esophagus connection) is located in the neck.

This procedure may also be considered minimally invasive as compared with the Ivor Lewis esophagectomy and the three incision esophagectomy.

How Far Back Do Esophagectomies Go?

The original esophagectomy was proposed in a lecture in 1946 by Ivor Lewis, which he gave at the Royal College of Surgeons in London. As originally described and implemented, this was a two-stage, two-day procedure.

---

[23] After my operation I was handed a paper with this healing track defined and explained. So each day I knew what was expected on my part to get out of the hospital. I was able to make it one day early!

The first stage consisted of a surgical incision into the abdominal cavity to loosen the stomach from the blood vessels, muscles, and tissue.

The second stage, performed ten to fifteen days later, was a surgical incision into the chest wall (thoracotomy) to loosen and remove the esophagus and then restructure the stomach into a new esophagus.

After that was completed, the surgeon would create an "anastomosis"—the connection which stapled the stomach and the remaining esophagus together to create the "new" esophagus in the throat.

Success Stats

Under Ivor Lewis, this operation was successful in five of seven patients, a tremendous feat for that era of medical practice. Over time this evolved into a single procedure, and today this type of operation continues to be used internationally and completed within six to eight hours in one day.

The advantages of this method include:

- excellent visualization of all parts of the operation;
- ability to perform two-field lymph node dissections;
- lower leak rate; and
- lower chance of injury to the recurrent laryngeal nerves.

The disadvantages include:

- the pain associated with a right thoracotomy,
- potential for higher respiratory complications, and

- increased toxicity if a leak occurs.[24]

Another Type of Esophagectomy

There is also a third technique besides the transhiatal and Ivor Lewis esophagectomy, called a "three incision esophagectomy." In this procedure the esophageal tumor is removed through an abdominal incision, right thoracic incision, and left neck incision. The anastomosis is again located in the neck.[25]

Which is Right for Me?

The type of esophagectomy chosen for someone would be doctor preference as well as patient factors. And perhaps some doctors are skilled in only one type or specialize in one type.

Asking which type would be used for your situation would enlighten you to the techniques and difficulties of the procedure as well as potential side effects.

When we first knew I had esophageal cancer and the word went out to friends, Dr. Alan Bloch, a friend from our University of Connecticut days, called me. He knew the protocol and that I was probably facing the complicated esophagectomy.

---

[24] "Open Ivor Lewis Esophagectomy" by Carolyn E. Reed, MD, *Science Direct*,
(http://www.sciencedirect.com/science/article/pii/S152229420900 0580).

[25] "Three Incision Esophagectomy," Stanford Health Care website,
(https://stanfordhealthcare.org/medical-treatments/e/esophagectomy.html).

He had one excellent piece of advice for me: "Dave, go to the best doctor you can find. This operation is complex, and it makes a difference who does it. Make sure they do a lot of these each year and that their 30-day post-op statistics are low!"

Here's the same advice found on the Stanford Health Care website: "The operation is technically challenging and can result in high mortality and morbidity if performed by less experienced surgeons who perform only a few esophagectomies per year."[26]

Since Alan was a doctor and had access to medical databases, he joined me in the search for the best doctor. Rather than going to an excellent surgeon on the East Coast, Midwest, or South, we discovered Dr. Oelschlager in Seattle.

He was an experienced surgeon in esophagectomies, doing them weekly, and he had less than a 1% mortality rate in the first thirty days after the operation. As I already mentioned, the national average is 9%.

This is opposed to another surgeon I found in the Northwest and with whom I consulted. I asked him what his thirty-day morbidity rate was, and I was shocked to learn it was 8%—one point less than the national average. He also did only a few operations each year instead of many surgeries.

I know this surgeon was a skillful, compassionate man and would have done the best he could in an operation. Perhaps it would have turned out as well as mine did with Dr. Oelschlager.

But doing my homework eliminated some "hope it goes well," which I couldn't afford in my situation, and guided

---

[26] Ibid.

me to an excellent, experienced surgeon in our region of the country. It also settled some angst in my mind.

Key Questions to Ask Your Potential Surgeon.

Alan also sent me this list of questions and other advice to assess the practicality of the operation and use in vetting a surgeon.

In re-reading my email, I've decided to add the whole piece here (with a couple edits) since it helped me so much to get beyond the "black hole" of the operation and settle me down emotionally. When a doctor speaks about how to deal with doctors, it's helpful.

For the past week, I have been reflecting some more on your situation and would like to share a few thoughts. First, I have several questions regarding your diagnostic evaluation (if you don't feel comfortable sharing this information, that's okay)

- What was the cell type (adenocarcinoma, squamous cell carcinoma, or something else)?

- Where was the tumor (how many centimeters from your incisor teeth during endoscopic examination)?

- What did the endoscopy report say?

- What did the pathology reports on the biopsies say?

- What did the CT scan report say?

- Was a PET scan done? (If so, what did the report say?)

- Was an esophageal ultrasound done? (If so, what did the report say?)

Second, I had some thoughts regarding your decision on whether to have surgery. In your decision-making process, it is important to weigh both the benefits and risks.

Regarding the benefits, according to your e-mail of January 19, you were given a 27%, 5-year survival probability with the chemo-radiation you received. With the addition of surgery, there was an additional 21% survival probability, bringing the total survival to nearly 50%.

A 5-year survival probability of 50% is pretty good for a diagnosis of esophageal cancer, considering many patients with esophageal cancer have a much lower survival rate due to more distant spread of the tumor. Moreover, patients with lung cancer or pancreatic cancer would be very envious to have a prognosis of a 50% five-year survival.

Regarding the risks, the most serious one is perioperative mortality, that is, mortality both during surgical hospitalization and after hospitalization.

Here is a web link to a recent review of esophageal cancer by Dr. Mark F. Berry, a thoracic surgeon who was at Duke and is now at Stanford: (http://www.ncbi.nlm.nih.gov/pmc/articles/PMC403 7413/#r73).

The article states that recent data from high-volume centers have shown low mortality rates of 1 % to 3.5%. However, studies involving population-based databases or multi-center trials show that esophageal resection continues to have relatively high perioperative mortality rates of 8.8% to 14%.

The conclusion from this is that you should consider having your surgery done at a high-volume center with a low mortality rate. Such centers have the best surgeons, the best operating room teams, and the best post-operative care. Because these centers see a lot of cases, they are very much at the top of their game.

Here are a few questions I would propose you consider asking a potential surgeon:

- How many patients with esophageal cancer has he operated on?

- How many patients a year with esophageal cancer has he operated on?

- What is the mortality rate during hospitalization? What complications have these patients had? Who is most at risk?

- What is the mortality rate after hospitalization? What complications have these patients had? Who is most at risk?

- What is the risk for someone in your physical condition?

- How many patients with Stage IIB (your stage??) esophageal cancer has he operated on?

- What is the 5-year survival rate for his patients with Stage IIB esophageal cancer?

- What surgeon would he go to if he needed surgery for esophageal cancer?

- Where would he go if he needed surgery for esophageal cancer?

- What are the high-volume centers in the country with the lowest mortality rates?

If I can end on a personal note, here's my thought: If I had the Stage IIB esophageal cancer, I would opt for surgery. But I would do it with the best surgeon I could find at the best institution I could find.

That way, I would have the best chance that the surgeon is able to remove all of the tumor, increasing my odds of long-term survival. And I would have the lowest risk of post-operative complications and death.

I hope this note is helpful in your decision-making process. I will keep you and Sheri in my prayers. Best wishes, Alan"

Personally, I'm always reluctant to treat a doctor as though they are on trial, but Alan assured me doctors are used to these types of questions and welcome them. If they don't graciously answer your questions, they either have bad bedside manners or you probably don't want to submit to them under the knife!

Needless to say, I was thankful for Alan's advice to find an excellent surgeon and how to vet them. I was also thankful to Alan for helping me overcome my reluctance to ask questions of my potential surgeon. The success of the operation totally affects my longevity on this planet.

Back to Dr. Oelschlager

The office door opened, and we found ourselves face-to-face with Dr. Brant Oelschlager and one of his interns. Dr. Oelschlager graciously answered my questions and explained more about what I would face in the operation and afterwards. This was a sobering conversation, highlighting again the morbid seriousness of esophageal cancer.

He ended the consultation by saying his assistant would call me to put an operation date on the calendar. We shook hands, said goodbye to them, and headed for the hospital car garage.

I knew making the decision would not be an easy one for me, so Sheri and I decided to spend a couple days on the Oregon Coast to process what lay ahead of us.

We found a small cottage on the beach and hunkered down to accomplish the objective, which was to decide: *To Operate or Not to Operate!*

My Decision About the Operation

Over those two days at the coast, I considered all the factors I knew in my situation (diagnosis, protocols, chemo-radiation results, advice, statistics, soul meditations I had written down, Sheri's and family member thoughts, Bible verses, etc.).

Coming out of that time, my decision was NOT to have the operation, but rather try to control and overcome any cancer still lurking in my body through naturopathic means (which are, in my mind, food, food supplements, juices, vitamin C infusions, and exercise).

Sheri and my children were in agreement with this, and I had the confidence (personal faith and confidence) to go down this road. So we committed ourselves to this path and planned our way forward.

Another Lesson Along the Way

What I learned through my experience is we each are unique individuals with unique cancer situations that must be treated in a unique way. We are each a "special case."

So the basic medical protocol is there, but this can be applied in many variations in each of our treatment paths.

And we are basically our own decision-makers for our health and life. Some of us in our uniqueness, defer quickly to the doctors and medical establishment in our decision-making.

Others of us do that after longer times of contemplation and deliberation. And some of us periodically decide to decline the medical advice and wisdom for other reasons.

The point is, we are each responsible for our own decisions and therefore cannot blame the hospital or doctor for the outcomes in our specific health situation.

And here's my "faith" statement I've added to the cancer protocol: Since God created each of us, He knows what's going on in our bodies and the reasons for that. If we look to Him for wisdom and insight about our cancer treatments just as we look to the doctors, He'll guide us into a good treatment path for us.

I love this statement of Israel's King David, which states this truth, "The LORD directs the steps of the godly. He delights in every detail of their lives" Psalm 37:23 (NLV).

5

DIVERSION FROM SURGERY...
HITTING CANCER WITH THE NATURAL!

Now that I had been successfully nuked, chemo-ed, and decided NOT to have the surgery, our path led us to the idea of using natural foods and supplements to deal with any remaining cancer cells existing in my body under the radar.

Remember, my statistic was that I had a 27% chance of making it to five years if I only did chemo-radiation. My chances of making it increased to 50% if I also did the operation.

This stat means, however, I would have a 73% chance of NOT making it to five years if I only stayed with chemo-radiation.

Isn't this just peaches and cream? Aren't stats just the thing you want to consider to make your day or your cancer decision?

So I had a choice to make with the stats: Did I want to be a pessimist and see the glass half empty? Or did I want to be an optimist and see the glass half full?

The pessimistic view was to camp on the fact I was in the 73% who wouldn't make it if I stopped now and didn't go on with surgery.

The optimistic view was to think I could actually be in the 27%. I mean, there are 27 of us out of 100 who ARE healed from the cancer through chemo-radiation alone! So which group would I visualize myself in and for what reasons?

Leaning Toward the Naturopathic

As I look back, I think it was all the encouragement of friends who had some experience with naturopathic medicine that stimulated our thinking in this direction. Then we started to do our own research and discovered the healing power of foods in the lives of others.

Sheri took the "research point" on all this data because it was of high interest to her. She is still a student of the natural healing track we continue with. I dove in a little as well. Based on our research, discussions between us, and credible friends, we decided to give the natural path a try.

After all, the rationale is quite logical, and natural remedies for sickness have been used from the beginning of time until today. In the western world, however, the influence of medical science in the twentieth century led to the establishment of the pharmaceutical industry which dominates us today and overshadows the natural.

I must acknowledge also that within naturopathic thinking, there are a lot of streams of thought and practices on the fringes I personally don't agree with. For example, in some literature and the teachings of some natural practitioners, the path starts out very much food oriented but then shifts into various meditations, mystical practices, new age-type thought, etc.

Personally, Sheri and I believe in using food for healing, but reject using that to move someone into a philosophical basket of mysticism. Life is full of sidetracks.

For us eating the right foods and using plants of the natural world to strengthen our immune systems, supplement our nutrition, and heal our bodies is naturopathic medicine. We're not interested in throwing out the baby with the bathwater. But we can't deny, there is some questionable bathwater.

What is the Naturopathic Theory?

The simple theory behind the natural treatment path is this: The body's immune system is capable of overcoming cancer most of the time. (Some naturopaths would say, "all of the time.") If we keep the immune system strong, it will ward off disease. (I guess that's why we always took some extra Vitamin C when a cold emerged.)

The problem is toxins in our environment and our foods wear down our immune system over a period of time. Once this happens, cancer and other diseases can take over without too much opposition from our suppressed immune system.

The solution is if we build up the immune system again, it will engage the bad cancer cells and overcome them.

Of course, there are other factors that play a part in killing cancer besides eliminating toxins, such as our DNA and stress levels. But the body is powerful, and the immune system has kept us healthy for many years from childhood into the teens, the twenties, etc.

So in our opinion, as we considered the essence of naturopathic medicine, this theory did not hit us as something "quacky," but resonated as truthful. What do you think? [27]

Naturopaths Painted as "Quacks"

Unfortunately, there's a latent and sometimes high-profile battle going on between the allopathic (established medical) community and the naturopathic community.

Our national history indicates the American Medical Association (AMA) and the USA pharmaceutical companies were able to gain the power differential over the naturopathic and homeopathic practitioners in the course of time in the early decades of the twentieth century.

During that formative time in our medical history, naturopaths were put out of business and painted as quacks and scammers. Some were undoubtedly quacks, as there are scammers in any profession today, including the established medical field. But most of the naturopaths we've met are conscientious professionals, as are our allopathic doctors and nurses.

As a result of this battle, many natural practitioners took their successful practices across the border to Mexico or Canada, and some medical centers still operate legally in these countries today, like the Gerson Center in Tijuana, Mexico.[28]

---

[27] "Naturopathy and the Primary Care Practice" by Sara A. Fleming and Nancy C. Gutknecht, PMC, USA National Library of Medicine, NIH, (https://www.ncbi.nlm.nih.gov/pmc/articles/PMC2883816/).

[28]The Gerson Institute Clinic in Tijuana, Mexico,

The Culture Wars

Here is a short description of the allopathic vs. naturopathic "wars" that took place in our medical history. I've taken this excerpt from a book report on Susan Catleff's book, *Nature's Path: A History of Naturopathic Healing in America*.

> One of the central themes of *Nature's Path* was the "culture wars" that raged between regular physicians (who became the American Medical Association in 1847) and the numerous alternative healing sects who opposed their methods and political heavy handedness.
>
> The centralized power of the AMA meant they controlled medical licensing, pharmaceuticals, public health authorities, police enforcement and military medicine. The government and major philanthropic foundations, through the AMA's powerful lobby, deemed only the allopathic (regular/AMA) physicians as credible and skilled.
>
> All others, regardless of their credentials and acquired knowledge could be, and were frequently, arrested for "practicing medicine without a license" under the plethora of medical licensing acts.[29]

(https://gerson.org/gerpress/gerson-clinic-mexico/). There are other types of medical clinics there as well. One I've used and can recommend is Dr. Isai Castillo's CIPAG Clinic, (http://www.drcastillo.com/).

[29] Interview with Susan E. Cayleff, Department of Women's Studies, San Diego State University. Posted on

Toward the end of the twentieth century, naturopathic medicine became more acceptable in spite of attempts to keep it on the back burner and without influence in the medical realm.

What most people don't know is that Naturopathic Doctors (NDs) actually have more academic medical training than the normal Medical Doctor (MDs). That's because they also study a huge amount of information about natural remedies to various illnesses.

Where the ND is more deficient in knowledge is in prescribing pharmaceuticals. Because the pharmaceutical companies put a lot of money into the allopathic track, MDs are well trained in which pill to use for which illness. Prescribing chemical medicine is the allopathic default for disease and illness.

The ND prefers not to use pharmaceuticals if at all possible and will prescribe natural products for disease and illness as their default.

For example, our naturopathic oncologist suggested we use blackberry syrup when sore throats start instead of some pill or pharmaceutical syrup. It's amazing what blackberry syrup will do. We haven't had a sore throat for three years! (Gargling with salt water is also a good natural remedy for a sore throat.)

If you are interested, there is an article that compares the training of Naturopathic Doctors (ND) with Medical Doctors (MD) in their first four years of training.[30]

(http://dailyhistory.org/Nature%27s_Path:_Interview_with_Susa n_E._Cayleff).

[30] Naturopathic Medicine Programs in the USA, from Association of Accredited Naturopathic Medical Colleges, (https://aanmc.org/resources/comparing-nd-md-curricula/).

Would Integrated Medicine be a Better Model Today?

According to some of the stalwarts in the naturopathic realm, the battle between some of the medical associations and naturopathic practice continues to this day.

Some laws favoring freedom to practice both types of medicine have been established. Yet a number of factions continue to skirt those laws today, pressuring naturopaths to stop their treatments.

If you are interested in more background, see the article by Dr. Joseph Mercola, who documents some of this continuing conflict.[31]

Dr. Mercola is an osteopathic physician, also known as a DO. DOs are licensed physicians who, similar to MDs, can prescribe medication and perform surgery in all fifty states. DOs and MDs have similar training, requiring four years of study in the basic and clinical sciences and the successful completion of licensing exams.

But DOs also practice a "whole person" approach and treat the entire person rather than mostly symptoms. They also focus on preventive health care, as do NDs.

Dr. Mercola is also board-certified in family medicine and served as chairman of the family medicine department at St. Alexius Medical Center for five years. He trained in both allopathic and naturopathic medicine.

Fortunately, many in the American allopathic profession today recognize the value of the naturopathic

---

[31] Posted December 13, 2011, on Dr. Joseph Mercola's website, "Chiropractors and Naturopaths—Are They Dangerous?" (http://articles.mercola.com/sites/articles/archive/2011/12/30/rethi nking-medical-associations-best-interests.aspx).

philosophy and are moving toward a more integrated model of treatment. Times are a changin', it seems.

For example, the Cleveland Clinic is one major medical institution taking a leadership role in the "integrative" direction. They provide a number of alternative treatments to what in the past has been considered the normal medical treatment track. Here's their description of alternative treatments:

> Cleveland Clinic's Center for Integrative and Lifestyle Medicine is dedicated to addressing the increasing demand for integrative healthcare by researching and providing access to practices that address the physical as well as lifestyle, emotional, and spiritual needs of patients. As the body of evidence for alternative medicine grows, we remain at the forefront providing the most up-to-date education and practices to patients. Cleveland Clinic's Center for Integrative and Lifestyle Medicine sees more than 5,000 patients per year for a variety of services.[32]

Here is the list of those naturopathic treatments they provide: nutrition, acupuncture, Chinese herbal medicine, chiropractic, culinary, energy, holistic psychotherapy, integrative, lifestyle, massage, nutrition, pain control, primary medicine, and yoga.

At the same time from the naturopathic side, many NDs are less antagonistic toward allopathic medicine and all the studies, statistics, and trials taking place in that realm.

---

[32] "Integrative and Lifestyle Medicine," Cleveland Clinic, (https://my.clevelandclinic.org/departments/wellness/integrative).

When we were looking for an ND in Bend, Oregon, after our natural treatments with Dr. Steve Morris in Mukilteo, Washington,[33] we found Dr. Katherine Neubauer in our town. Not only is she a trained ND, but she also has a specialty in oncology. She is one of the seventy trained naturopathic oncologists in the USA!

She treats us with natural supplements and products and coordinates with Dr. Martin, our oncologist, to know what treatments and advice he is giving us. Her advice is normally based on cancer studies being done with specific natural products.[34]

For example, in Germany they discovered that mistletoe is a good, natural, anti-cancer treatment. So three times each week, I injected mistletoe serum imported from Germany.

Dr. Neubauer uses an integrated approach, and Dr. Martin's Center, the St. Charles Cancer Center, in Bend, Oregon, is starting to branch out into some alternative treatments like nutrition, massage, and yoga.

Unfortunately, not every doctor or institution in the USA is as open and forward-looking as these two doctors, the St. Charles Cancer Center, or Cleveland Clinic are.

For example, a friend of ours was recently diagnosed with Stage III colon cancer. At the time, she decided against the allopathic protocol recommended by her doctor (chemo, radiation, and operation), so she could try naturopathic treatments for a period of time, similar to what I have done.

---

[33] "Mukilteo Natural Health Clinic," Mukilteo, Washington, (http://www.mukilteonaturalhealth.com/profile/other/steve-morris/).

[34] "Cascade Cancer Care," Bend, Oregon, (http://www.cascadecancercare.com/about/about-us/).

After only a couple weeks on naturopathic treatments, she passed a tissue lump and asked her medical doctor to lab test it for cancer. Many on naturopathic treatments have had tumors expelled from their bodies through the bowels, mouth, or skin. She wondered if this was her case. She also asked for an MRI.

Her medical doctor refused both requests because she had not followed the protocol!

Her naturopath was able to request an MRI, but in today's American medical world, the insurance companies do not pay for naturopathic treatments except chiropractic. So our friend had to pay for this expense herself—an out-of-pocket cost of $600.

How quickly the integrated approach will be accepted by either camp is still an open question. I personally hope ego, ignorance, and bias are all put aside for the patient's good.

At the moment the allopathic establishment has the power in our society since the insurance and pharmaceutical companies back them with their research and dollars.

Fortunately, most naturopathic treatments are available in the USA today with the financial caveat I already alluded to: If we want them, we must cover these costs out of our own pockets because the insurance industry won't cover them.

While there's actually no comparison in prices—one chemo treatment can cost the insurance company $40,000, and a three-week anti-cancer naturopathic treatment can cost $9,000—the naturopathic treatment cost must be borne by the patient. On fixed budgets like most of us have, this is hard to bear.

Of course, while the critics of naturopathic medicine will agree with the pricing comparison, they might say the disparity is because of effectiveness. Their contention is that allopathic methods are more effective.

Unfortunately effectiveness cannot be measured because there are no studies being done to compare allopathic apples with naturopathic apples. So we are left with bias, hearsay, and innuendo on all sides.

And with the medical industry's research dollars going to the allopathic track, it doesn't appear we'll get those comparative studies anytime soon.

This means individual American citizens are the ones who suffer from fewer treatment choices unless they have the financial ability to pay for these as extra costs. Not all of us can!

Natural Treatment Lesson

One thing we noticed about our natural treatments is they built up our immune systems and carried us on a higher health level INTO our medical treatments.

For example, since our start of these natural products and better food in February 2015, neither of us has had a cold, sore throat, or the flu into December 2017, at the time of this publishing. And last year we had a cold, hard winter in Central Oregon!

Sheri's Experience

Sheri had two bouts with lymphoma cancer. In 2010—pre-natural treatments—she faced a fast-growing tumor, knocked out by a five-month chemo regimen. During this time, she was very sick with nausea and sat in her chair most of the time resting. Basically, she was immobilized by the chemo treatments and feeling sick.

Fortunately, we had an "angel" appear to provide food for us (since my cooking ability relates to scalding the water, and burning the corn flakes). Our good Samaritan friend had a personal goal to keep us in food from the first day of treatment until Sheri was back on her feet after the last one! She thankfully accomplished that goal, and we ate very well! *Thank you, Georgia!*

The second time Sheri faced off against cancer was 2015—mid-stream during our natural treatments—when a slow-growing lymphoma tumor showed up on the radar screen.

She was just about to her five-year remission date—the major cancer remission marker—when this showed up on the CT scan and had to be treated. So once again Sheri decided to take the recommended chemo to knock the tumor down.

Granted the chemo was different than the first time and perhaps a little milder, but during these chemo treatments she was able to continue operating a normal schedule and carry out her daily tasks, including cooking! She was her own angel this time.

During this second fight with cancer, she would have a couple "down days" 48-72 hours after each treatment. But otherwise she operated her life as normal since her body and immune system were very strong.

She believes the strength of her immune system got her through the tough chemo infusions better the second time than the first time. This is because she was strengthened with naturopathic treatments prior to taking the chemo as well as concurrently with the chemo regimen.

In an integrated way, both of these treatments were coordinated between Dr. Martin and Dr. Neubauer as she went along.

<u>My Experience</u>

I had the same experience with my esophagectomy. I went into this operation being at peak immune system performance with excellent metrics, like blood tests. I also attribute this to the naturopathic principles we've applied in our eating, supplements, and exercise for the two years prior to my operation.

So here's our advice: If you are heading into chemo treatments or operations of any type, "natural up" the body's immune system prior to your procedure, possibly during your procedure, and again after the treatment.

I say, "perhaps during your procedure" because that phase particularly should be done in consultation with your doctor. In operations, your doctor is concerned about blood coagulation count to ensure against abnormal bleeding. Often pills as well as supplements could affect the blood coagulation time and/or perhaps hinder chemo effectiveness in some way. So it's best practice to keep your doctors informed in order to apply an integrated form of medicine.

How We Implemented Our "Natural Treatment" Decision

As I mentioned, Sheri discovered her second lymphoma tumor in December 2014, just before I finished my radiation treatments on January 6, 2015.

So after we made the decision to treat my esophageal cancer with naturopathic means and her lymphoma naturopathically as well, the issue was where do we go to get moving with this?

Some friends of ours recommended a friend of theirs, Dr. Steve Morris,[35] an ND in Mukilteo, Washington. We contacted him and were able to get a consultation. Through that discussion, we felt he could help us with both of our cancer situations.

Dr. Morris suggested we take four weeks of treatment, five mornings a week. For that period of time, another friend offered us the use of their cottage on Whidbey Island free of charge. So we were ready to give this healing path a try.

Then to put the icing on the cake, a cousin of Sheri's gave us the money to pay for all these extra treatments since our insurance didn't cover any of them. This was no small expense, but a very generous gift to us and our health.

The Cost of Naturopathic Treatments

As I mentioned above, natural treatments are not cheap because they are out-of-pocket expenses to the patient. Most insurance policies and Medicare do not pay to provide natural treatments for these reasons:

1) Naturopathic medicine has been marginalized in the US as we saw above, and is, therefore, suspect concerning effectiveness.
2) Naturopathic clinical trials have little financial backing because the money for these trials flows through and from the pharmaceutical industry. This industry is a profit-based, bottom-line controlled conglomerate with strong lobbying efforts in Washington. Today the money is made in promoting and using chemical drugs.

---

[35] http://www.mukilteonaturalhealth.com/.

3) Naturopathic products don't create much money since they are, well, natural. For example, there is simply not much money to be made harvesting mistletoe from a tree and making that into a product, whereas the development of Lipitor returns billions.[36]

And patents are more difficult to gain on a natural plant (although the US government does have a patent on the marijuana plant).[37]

It's unfortunate this divide between allopathic and naturopathic medicine exists today. I'm not sure what would change the practice of the insurance industry, but at the moment only a few insurance companies provide money for only a few naturopathic treatments even though many of the treatments are preventive and would most likely cost the industry less money in the long run. Healthy people don't cost their health insurance company money!

For example, I have not been to my general MD for three years because I've been in an out of my oncologist's office during that time. He gave me blood tests and kept track of my heart and lungs. So I felt I didn't need my general MD. Nothing popped up of a negative health nature during that time besides tracking on my cancer.

---

[36] Description of Lipitor, a cholesterol lowering drug, (http://www.lipitor.com/about).

[37] These articles in *The Denver Post* and *The Cannabist* give background on the US Government's marijuana patent and some of the issues involved:
(http://www.denverpost.com/2016/08/28/what-is-marijuana-patent-6630507/),
(http://www.thecannabist.co/2016/08/22/marijuana-patents-6630507-research-dea-nih-fda-kannalife/61255/).

So my MDs office finally called me and asked, "Are you still wanting to be a patient of ours?" Of course, I didn't want to lose my general practitioner who is an excellent doctor, so I went in for a check-up and talk.

In hindsight it would have been wise for me to keep up with an annual- or eighteen-month checkup because my general doctor is tracking on my overall health condition. He has the overview none of my specialists have.

However, my point is, other than the cancer, I've been so healthy I didn't need my general doctor to treat anything else in my overall health. So my insurance company saved their money. I attribute that to the natural medical track we've been on.

Back to Our Treatments …

We took the car ferry over to Whidbey Island and moved into our friend's cottage. Five days a week we hiked a mile over to the ferry and sailed back and forth across the channel between Whidbey and Mukilteo. Feet and ferry were a healthy transportation for us while doing healthy treatments! And spotting some orcas in the channel was always delightful.

The first step Dr. Morris took with us was to shift our eating patterns from a high meat, carb, and sugar diet to a vegetarian one—not an easy task for someone who, from childhood on, ate a typical daily Dutch diet of meat, potatoes, vegetables, and heavy dessert.

The second step was to make five juices a day. These alternated between fruit smoothies and vegetable juices with lots of greens, ginger, and turmeric root. Every two hours starting in the afternoon when we arrived back at the cottage, we were in the kitchen blending and then consuming our sometimes-tasty juices.

The third step was for us to have a vitamin-C infusion each morning. So 25ml of that vitamin in liquid form was pumped into our veins as we sat in Dr. Morris' infusion room. Several other patients would also be there for various infusions and treatments, and some interesting conversations ensued on contrails, natural medicine, cancer, spiritual life, and food.

In addition to infusions, Dr. Morris also prescribed a variety of supplements we took each day. And we had a consultation with him each week to ensure progress and gain answers to our questions. Slowly we were being educated in naturopathic thinking and practice.

The fourth step was our introduction to the Gerson coffee enema treatment. A German doctor, Max Gerson, developed this treatment in the 1940s as part of his natural anti-cancer protocol. The scientific rationale and value for this therapy, as well as a one-page bio on Dr. Gerson, is found in Appendix B.[38]

Fred Meyer produced the enema bags; Whole Foods produced the organic mild coffee to be used; our coffee pot produced the hot, brewed coffee; our behinds produced the location; and we were off and running with this therapy!

Buying Natural and Organic

In Mukilteo we located the Whole Foods organic store about ten miles away and made regular treks there to purchase all of our organic fruits and vegetables. As tough as it was for me initially, I disciplined myself to walk past

---

[38] Dr. Max Gerson and the Gerson Institute, (https://gerson.org/gerpress/dr-max-gerson/).

the meat counter where the steak beckoned and look the other way at checkout where the candy bars enticed!

Their hot food buffet was always delicious, however. So a diversion was to take our delectables from there when getting our groceries.

Other restaurant visits were very limited—most don't serve organic food, and vegetarian dishes are normally not on the menu. We found a local Chinese Restaurant, however, that did have a vegetarian dish, or we could "special order" one. Going out for dinner kept us feeling normal as we adjusted to a new way of thinking about diet and changing our actual eating habits.

So this was our life for one month as we switched from our heavy red-meat diet to a vegetarian one. Dr. Morris recommended we stay on a vegetarian diet but said we could also bring in some meat later if we liked. With a smile on his face, he said, "You can have a yearly steak!" (Actually, I haven't had any steak since my operation seven months ago, since chunks of beef still don't look good to me. I am finally eating ground beef again; so I think my healing is progressing.)

Later on, Dr. Neubauer suggested it would be wise to have more protein in our diet. She recommended we include some chicken and fish along with our heavy vegetable diet.

We wrapped up our time with Dr. Morris, his son, Aaron, also an ND, and their staff. We packed up, cleaned the cottage and headed back around the bend to Bend, Oregon…Happy Cottage Campers, feeling great!

We were feeling so good, our inner question was, "Do we really have cancer?"

Continuing Our Naturopathic Journey Back Home

One loose end we needed to tie up after leaving Dr. Morris was to find a naturopath in Bend to continue our treatments. Our research led us to Dr. Katherine Neubauer, whom I already mentioned and who had just arrived in Bend to set up her practice. We were fortunate to find her in our little town.

Dr. Neubauer[39] is one of only sixty-two hospital-trained, board-certified, oncology naturopaths in the USA. She comes from a long line of doctors in her family working to defeat cancer.

Her great uncle, Dr. Sidney Farber, founded modern chemotherapy as well as the Dana Farber Cancer Institute at Harvard University. Her grandfather, Dr. Seymour Farber, discovered how smoking tobacco causes cancer. Together they worked in the 'War on Cancer' and hoped and believed that war could be won.

Then cancer hit very close to home for Dr. Neubauer. Her other grandfather got lung cancer, and her grandmother got breast cancer. They followed the best treatment protocols available at the time, which killed the cancer cells but devastated their health. When the cancer came back they were too ill and weak to fight.

That background and those experiences led Dr. Neubauer to join the search for a better way to eliminate cancer. This led her from her allopathic medical studies into the area of natural healing as well. Today she combines both

---

[39] This biographical information is taken from Dr. Neubauer's website: (https://www.cascadecancercare.com).

approaches in her treatment of patients in an integrated way.

We had our initial consultations with her and entered into treatment. Besides some additional or other supplements, she added the mistletoe injections for me.

Sheri and I both continued our weekly Vitamin C infusions, but Dr. Payton Flattery,[40] another ND in Bend, who owns the lab where we had our infusions, kicked up the amount of our vitamin C infusion liquid from 25ml to 50ml.

When we arrived back in Bend, Sheri, under Dr. Martin's care, also headed into her second round of chemo treatments against the slow-growing lymphoma. I spent much of my time enjoying life and writing a major resource to help international workers fund their work. Life was more or less back to normal.

Dr. Martin agreed to monitor my cancer via blood tests. So I put off having any more scans in order to reduce the nuclear footprint in my body.

Sheri beat her cancer over the next few months through her chemo treatment augmented by continued natural treatment. Her last CT scan showed absolutely no lymphoma on the screen. She was officially in remission.

I felt wonderful and proceeded on in good health and with quality of life…for another year and a half…until I had a PET scan to establish a new baseline for my tumor. The eclipse continues…

---

[40] Dr. Flattery has an established naturopathic practice in Bend, Oregon, (http://centerforintegratedmed.com/integrative-medicine/practitioners/payson-flattery-nd-dc-daapm/).

6
THE NATURAL...NOT ENOUGH!

After a year and nine months of treating my cancer through natural means, while observing my blood test numbers every three months (always excellent), Dr. Martin suggested I do a PET scan again to create a new monitoring baseline. This would ensure the cancer was not growing or spreading.

So I dutifully, and in full agreement with his logic, headed over to Central Oregon Radiology Associates to take on the PET scan.

PETS, PETS, and More PETS (And I don't mean your dog!)

PET stands for "positron emission tomography." A PET scan is a procedure designed to identify abnormal cellular activity that might indicate cancer. A prominent use for the PET scan (or combination PET/CT) is in achieving accurate staging of cancer by identifying the extent of its growth.

In a PET scan, the patient is injected with a glucose-based tracer substance: think of it as hot sugar. The PET scan picks up where this "sugar" localizes in the body.

The idea applied to oncology is that the cancer cells, because they're very active, eat up more sugar than non-cancerous cells. Therefore, the cancer cells will collect this tracer, resulting in a brighter appearance in those cells on the scan than in normal tissue cells. (Now you know why I try to limit my sugar intake as I fight cancer! I hear the cancer cells crying out, "Feed me! Feed me!")

When my PET results came back, I breathed a sigh of relief. The good news was the cancer tumor had not metastasized. The bad news was the intensity of the tumor had increased, which indicated higher cancer cell activity.

This was measured by a metric called "SUV."

SUV—Not Your "Sport Utility Vehicle!"

PET scan results are reported in "SUV" units as well as other metrics. SUV does not stand for "sport utility vehicle," but rather for "standardized uptake value." The SUV is a measurement indicating how bright the tissue is on the PET scan; that is, how intense the cellular activity is occurring in that area.

This activity however, is not only cancer specific, but can represent other damaged cell issues varying from inflammation to infection to cancer.

The fact is, there is no threshold SUV number that distinguishes cancer from inflammation or infection, but higher numbers (especially in the high single digits or more) are most suggestive of cancer.

A factor of 2.5 indicates the benign standard although this again is not an exact scientific measurement.

In my case, because cancer had been diagnosed before, my SUV readings were definitely a marker of cancer activity. Cancer cells were identified in the tumor through my endoscopic biopsy in 2014 and simply verified by the SUV metric from my PET scans.

As you see from my numbers below, the intensity of the tumor was on the incline. (I never did ask if this was an inflammation increase, growth of cells increase, or another factor. I should have become more knowledgeable on this factor early on!)

1) October 03, 2014—SUV 6.25. This was my marker in my first PET scan diagnosing my cancer.

2) January 26, 2015—SUV 3.86. Indicated some minor activity after my chemo-radiation treatments. But since my tests were taken close to the end of radiation, we could not tell if the cancer activity would decline or continue to incline. We decided to track activity with blood tests.

3) September 16, 2016—SUV 13.0 Charting this increase meant the intensity of cell activity was doubling every year, and would eventually metastasize. This test was eighteen months from the end of radiation.

4) December 05, 2016—SUV 15.2. This PET scan was taken after my treatment in Mexico, which I'll describe later. This scan showed positive results in tumor size but with lack of metastasis. It also highlighted an increased cell activity within the tumor. This increase was in line with the one-year doubling metric.

So based on the December 5 scan, I made the decision to have the tumor taken out, and this is how that happened!

Hit the Home Run!

In my consultation with Dr. Martin to go over the results of my third PET scan, the September 16, 2016, scan, we talked again about having the operation. He suggested I was still a candidate for the surgery since the cancer had not yet metastasized.

Using a baseball analogy, he said, "Perhaps you'll hit the home run and be cured!" I didn't like the word "perhaps" since I knew my batting average was not like Babe Ruth's, who usually hit a home run. (In the days before drugs enhanced natural power!)

Even though I could see the handwriting on the wall concerning cancer growth, I was still not in a personal and emotional space to say "yes" to the operation. (What's wrong with me, right? Is my head in the sand like the ostrich?)

At the same time, however, we knew the natural treatments to-date were not powerful enough to turn the cancer totally back.

We could confidently say natural treatments had dampened its progress and gave me some modicum of control over the cancer. But it seemed the tumor was too large of a mass for my present attempts to stop it by natural means.

Another option was to try and nail the tumor with a more "high-powered" natural treatment than I was presently using.

Dr. Neubauer, in a consultation at this time, verified she had no studies in naturopathic medicine where an esophageal tumor was totally healed through natural treatments. Somehow that piece of vital info didn't register in my brain before as I started naturopathic treatments.

However, that knowledge probably wouldn't have changed my disposition at the time anyway because of my negative view of the operation.

Because of factors already mentioned in this book, I was aware there simply weren't a lot of studies in naturopathic medicine. So my thought about having another heavy naturopathic treatment was, "Naturopathic medicine cannot be discounted as healing esophageal cancer, but we don't have a record it's ever happened."

I realized my choices were very limited. If I continued on the same path of dealing with my cancer, the best result would be palliative care and my demise quicker than I had hoped.

At some point in the not too distant future, the cancer would metastasize into my lymph system and organs. And without another endoscopy, I simply didn't know how close the tumor was to eating through the two outside layers of my esophagus to create that result.

Let's Head for Mexico!

So now I had to make another decision: Do I put the operation into motion, or hit the cancer harder with natural treatments?

A friend of ours living in San Diego, Yvonne, was diagnosed with breast cancer thirty years ago. Rather than have chemo and a potential operation at that time, she and her husband discovered Dr. Isai Castillo and his CIPAG Clinic just across the border in Tijuana, Mexico. He was treating cancer with mostly natural means although he can be integrative in his approach as well. Mexico has more freedom in all types of treatment options than we do in the USA.

Yvonne started Dr. Castillo's treatments, and after completion of those over a period of a couple years, she was cancer free and has maintained that for the past thirty years.

When she and her husband heard of my dilemma, they wrote me to consider Dr. Castillo's clinic for my natural cancer treatments. They sweetened the suggestion by their offer to use their home if we came, since they would be on a trip and gone while we were there.

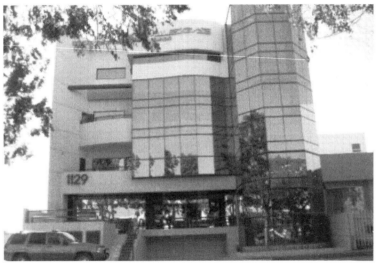

The CIPAG Clinic Building

To do my homework, I called Dr. Castillo and discussed the possibility of his treatments. He could take me as a patient during the twenty-one days I wanted. He informed me the cost would be between $7,000 and $9,000 depending on the extent of my treatments. Some treatments were the basic regimen. Others were special ones based on specific disease factors and prescribed as the treatment progressed.

After gaining this information, we checked our piggy bank and a couple of other options for funding this. Isn't life interesting? We give up our health to create money so we can retire. Then when we retire we use our money to get our health back! Anything wrong with this picture?

We discussed this option further, gained some counsel, prayed over this direction, and finally made the decision to go for it, putting the operation on hold for a second time.

After Dr. Martin and Dr. Neubauer were informed of our decision, we packed up our Toyota and took off for San Diego!

Are Mexican Clinics a Good Alternative Option?

When the subject of Mexican clinics comes up, there are a host of pros and cons that also surface depending on who you talk with. For example, one says, "They are effective, and many have been helped," while another says, "They scam you, have killed people, and use crazy treatments."

I know you can probably find examples on both of these perspectives. So what are the objective and solid facts we can say about alternative treatment in a Mexican clinic? Here are my opinions from limited experience.

There are a number of clinics in Mexico catering to *gringos,* although many citizens of Mexico use them as well. One article said at least thirty-eight clinics exist in Tijuana alone. And there are other border towns with more.

It's very possible a few of these clinics could be fraudulent in some way. "The love of money is the root of all evil" is an international phenomenon. It has no respect for borders since it's carried in the heart of man.

So, how do we sort out the good from the bad without claiming all of them are illegitimate? That seems to be a valid question.

There are at least two ways to sort out the legitimate from the illegitimate in my perspective. Either we receive a good recommendation from someone we trust, or we do some research into the credibility of any clinic we're considering for alternative treatment.

A good source for research on foreign alternative medicine clinics is Ralph Moses. He has been researching these clinics and writing about them for a number of years. He also gives personal consultations and has info on his website: (http://cancerdecisions.com).

In my general research and experience here's what I found:

- *Mexico allows some treatments the USA has banned.* However, it's wise to ask the question why some substance or treatment was banned here. In my research on the banning of the Hoxsey tonic, for example, the reason looks more political, economic, and ego driven rather than product-danger driven. (I've used this tonic for some time, and I'm healthy!) So we need to consider what "behind the scenes" agendas are either promoting or degrading treatments offered by Mexican clinics.

- *Many of the patients going to the Mexican clinics are in Stage IV cancer situations.* The medical establishment somewhere has "cut these patients loose" because they can't do more for them through medical means. While at CIPAG, we met one American and several Canadians in this situation.

If patients go to a Mexican clinic in this desperate condition, some will be helped while others might die. There is anecdotal evidence for that fact. But is it right to condemn clinics in Mexico for deaths when they are trying to help people with Stage IV cancer survive longer—

especially when the medical establishment isn't able to help them?

- *The stories of people being helped and healed through Mexican clinics is anecdotal* without studies being done to prove treatments actually work. We must keep in mind, however, that it takes money to do studies.

The Mexican government is not allocating funds for studies. And neither the American pharmaceutical companies nor our government are allocating funds for naturopathic research either.

So plants, juices, supplements, tonics, etc., may be very effective treatments, but we don't know it and can't scientifically prove it.

The critique seems to go like this: Someone healed in this way creates an anecdote, while someone who dies, creates proof the treatment is false. Is that a fair way to handle this issue?

Where Does All the Research Money Go Anyway?

While we're in an analysis mode, there's one more issue we should consider. Since not much research money is going toward naturopathic medicine, what impact is the money having on the allopathic track (which includes big pharma), especially on cancer research.

Because we're especially interested in the cancer side of the equation, we could ask, "Where does all our cancer research money go, and what's it accomplishing?"

Dr. David Chan, oncologist, said in *Quora Digest*:

I'll be the first to admit that despite all the billions put into cancer research, the end results of preventing cancer and treating advanced cancer have been disappointing.

Unlike reducing deaths from heart attacks and stroke, progress in reducing deaths from cancer has been disappointingly slow. Sure, we've had our breakthrough drugs like Gleevec, the targeted drug for chronic myelogenous leukemia, and Herceptin, for a certain type of breast cancer.[41]

But for a lot of other cancers, the treatments aren't giving us bang for the buck. Spending $100,000 to $200,000 a year to extend life for an additional three to six months may be very important to those individuals with cancer, but is a very poor return on investment for society.[42]

In the same article, Dr. Margaret Cuomo (sister of New York governor, Andrew Cuomo) is quoted from her perspective in her recent book, *A World Without Cancer*:

More than forty years after the war on cancer was declared, we have spent billions fighting the good fight. The National Cancer Institute has spent some $90 billion on research and treatment during that time. Some 260 nonprofit organizations in the USA have dedicated themselves to fight cancer—more than the number established for heart disease, AIDS, Alzheimer's disease, and stroke combined. Together,

---

[41] Herceptin was also effective for my 'morphed' esophageal cancer type. The third endoscopic biopsy determined this.

[42] Article by Dr. David Chan, M.D. in *Quora Digest*, "Where do the Millions of Cancer Research Dollars Go Every Year?" (http://www.slate.com/blogs/quora/2013/02/07/where_do_the_m illions_of_cancer_research_dollars_go_every_year.html).

these 260 organizations have budgets that topped $2.2 billion in 2013.

It's true there have been small declines in some common cancers since the early 1990s, including male lung cancer, colon, and rectal cancer in both men and women. And the fall in the cancer death rate—by approximately 1% a year since 1990—has been slightly more impressive. Still, that's hardly cause for celebration. Cancer's role in one out of every four deaths in this country remains a haunting statistic.[43]

Wouldn't it be nice to reach the point in integrative medicine when the insurance company or American government would allow the patient to make the decision about what type of treatment they want in a given year— for example the 10K treatment for cancer by an approved Mexican or German clinic or the 200K chemo treatment in an American cancer center?

It would seem some accommodation like this could be reached—except for governmental, allopathic, and pharmaceutical bias against naturopathic medicine.

A Good Time in Mexico

What a lovely time we had in San Diego, basing our visit out of our friends' home. Six days a week for three weeks, we drove back and forth across the Mexican border— fortunately going the opposite direction of rush hour traffic

---

[43] Dr. Margaret Cuomo quote from an article by Dr. David Chan in *Quora Digest*,
(http://www.slate.com/blogs/quora/2013/02/07/where_do_the_m illions_of_cancer_research_dollars_go_every_year.html).

in San Diego. Thus, we missed the freeway parking lots stretching for miles each way at certain times of the day!

The first day, we zipped across the border going in, but coming out took us over an hour of waiting for US customs to clear us.

After the first day, we found the "medical line" coming out, but that still took about an hour of waiting before reaching our customs agents, with their stern-faced questioning. Our clinic's letter of intent and the "infusion bandage" on my arm helped confirm our reason for being in Mexico—medical treatments at CIPAG.

Dr. Castillo and his staff are located in a modern building only five minutes away from the Mexican-US border. The first day, as we followed the directions from the clinic's website, we missed the road but soon happened on it again without getting too lost.

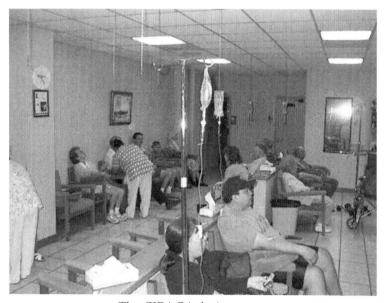

The CIPAG infusion room

The staff was very friendly and helpful, as were the group of patients being treated, many from Canada. One outgoing Canadian couple warmly welcomed us as we sat in the hallway chatting and waiting for my turn for a place in the infusion room. (It was on a first-come, first-served basis, so get there early!)

I started my treatment with blood tests, another CT scan, and a consultation with Dr. Castillo and Dr. Espanoza. My PET scans and blood tests from Bend were sent via email before we arrived, so they had that data already

A required trip to their in-house pharmacy netted us a list of supplements to take as well as the Hoxsey Tonic—an anti-cancer liquid developed by John Hoxsey and his son, Harry, veterinarians who were put out of business by the AMA.[44]

Eliminating Twenty Cancer Soldiers!

My weekly consultations with one of the three doctors in the clinic, alongside the infusions, were always enjoyable and enlightening.

In one of those consultations with Dr. Espinoza, a Mexican ND trained at Loma Linda University in the USA, I asked the question, "What counsel can you give me about having the esophagectomy if these treatments don't slow down the cancer and eliminate it?"

I was not expecting his answer because he replied to my question with his own question, "Dave, if you want to fight

---

[44] "History of Hoxsey Treatment" by Patrician Ward Spain, (http://www.tldp.com/issue/166/166hoxs.htm).
This is a short summary of the conflict between Fishbein (AMA) and Hoxsey, as well as studies regarding the Hoxsey Tonic and verification of many of the ingredients in it.

a battle, would you rather do that against twenty soldiers or against five?"

Unless someone is feeling like Superman—and after all my infusions I was feeling quite good, but not that good! — the answer is obvious: It's better to take on five soldiers rather than twenty. In any battle, the objective is to win, but at a minimum, you at least want to survive!

The application of Dr. Espanoza's illustration for me was obvious. The twenty soldiers I was fighting was the massive esophageal tumor still in my body, still kicking up with some level of intensity, and not yet ready for death without taking me there at the same time.

The tumor battle had been going on for almost three years. My blood tests indicated I was on the winning track. But the PET scans indicated the cells were growing and still had strength. How to win the battle?

An option was to have the esophagectomy and knock out at least fifteen, if not all, of the soldiers. After that I could use whatever means available to take on the five soldiers that were left if, in fact, any were left.

Or the possibility still existed with the operation that I could gain the exceptional result expressed in this mixed metaphor: "I could hit the home run and knock out the twenty soldiers in one battle with the operation."

Dr. Espinoza's thought was the first time and the first concept about the operation I heard, that made sense to me. Or perhaps I had processed this for so long, I was now emotionally and practically open to the operation?

I pondered this. I discussed it with Sheri. I prayed about it. And I decided if the Mexican clinic treatments did not knock the cancer back in a major way, showing I was on the upward winning track, I would submit to the operation.

In the final few days of treatments, I ended my time in Mexico with another CT scan, blood test, and final consultation with Dr. Castillo. My blood tests were still sterling, prompting Dr. Castillo to say, "I wish I had those numbers for my blood."

I was feeling great. My immune system was chugging along at 100%. Would I defeat the cancer in this natural way or not?

On our trip home we booked a room in a hotel on the beautiful Southern California coast for a few days and then drove the next two days home to Bend, Oregon. Fall colors graced our way, especially around the area of Redding, California. We were upbeat and optimistic. The darkness had now been eclipsed again with some light.

Before I would decide about the operation, I needed to wait two months to have another PET scan. Would the Mexico treatments work in my case or not? That was the $64,000 question.

PET Scan Results Directed My Decision

In December 2016, after waiting those two months and following the daily protocol of treatments prescribed by Dr. Castillo, I had my PET scan.

Sitting in Dr. Martin's office, we discussed the results. The cancer had intensified via the SUV marker from 13.0 to 15.2. The Mexico treatments had not held it in check or reversed the trajectory.

Dr. Castillo had indicated two months of waiting would be the earliest I should get the PET scan. So it's possible if I had another month or two before the PET scan, the SUV marker might have declined.

I will never know if that was the case or not since I decided not to wait any longer to take on the twenty soldiers and try to knock them out—and hit the home run at the same time!

I was finally emotionally, practically, intellectually, and spiritually ready for the operation.

But now, was it still feasible, or had the cancer metastasized and eliminated that possibility? And would Dr. Oelschlager still be willing to do the operation since I turned him down two times before?

7

OUT IT COMES—THE TRANSHIATAL ESOPHAGECTOMY!

Since I was processing all along the way, it was not a major decision to have the operation once the picture of the soldiers fixated in my mind and heart. My decision hinged on the SUV reading of the last PET scan. When that indicated an increase of 2.2 in a little over two months, my decision was made.

The PET scan at that time still indicated no metastasis. So as far as Dr. Martin was concerned, the operation was a "green light" for the procedure he had recommended from the start.

Choosing the Best Doctor for You

I've already shared thoughts about finding the best doctor you can for such a complicated operation. On a scale of 1-10, 10 being the most difficult, the esophagectomy is most likely a 9.

Basically, in this operation, they are re-sectioning your innards, giving you a new esophagus by reforming your stomach. Normally it takes two doctors to perform a successful operation, so choosing the best overall surgeon for the task (who then chooses his second in command) is the excellent way to go.

Since I had already consulted with Dr. Brant Oelschlager once before, and because I felt he was the most excellent thoracic surgeon in the Northwest for me, I set up another consultation with him.

My critical question for him was: Since you agreed to do the operation two years ago, and I turned it down, are you still willing to do the operation for me now?

We set up an appointment with him again at the University of Washington Medical Center in Seattle, and we drove the six hours from Central Oregon for another consultation. Actually, we broke up the trip for a fun diversion on the way to Seattle by stopping in Leavenworth, Washington.

A Personal "Rabbit Trail" Regarding Leavenworth

Because we spent fourteen years living in beautiful Austria and one year in the Black Forest region of Germany, we gained a love for the German countries and culture. Leavenworth is a "German" town—not by ancestry, but by design.

In the 1960s the lumber industry in the Northwest United States was being shut down. Environmental groups were putting on pressure to save the forests and using the spotted owl as their tool to stop logging.

It worked. The lumber towns across Oregon and Washington ground to a halt. Lumber mills closed, and small, thriving lumber towns were put out of business. Leavenworth was one of those.

Humor from those Times

A lumber mill in Oregon was shut down due to the spotted owl lobbying. All the workers were now out of a job. A logger with four children in Central Oregon was one of those laid off.

Often his children and wife would be hungry, and he had no money to feed them. So he would hunt to provide their food. One night he noticed a spotted owl in a tree, got out his shotgun, fired off a round, and provided food for his family that night.

Unfortunately, it's illegal to kill spotted owls, and the game warden found out he did that. He was hauled into court before the judge.

The judge asked him, "Sir, did you actually kill a spotted owl?"

"Yes," he replied, "But could I explain the extenuating circumstances?"

"Go ahead," the judge said.

So the man continued, "Judge, I've got four kids and a wife. When the green lobby shut down the mill, I was out of work. Yet I had to provide for my family. So one night I saw the spotted owl in a pine tree on my property and shot it to provide food for my family."

The judge said, "Okay. I understand. Because of your circumstances, I'm going to let you go this time. We probably won't miss one owl anyway. Just don't do it again."

As the man was going out of the courtroom thankful for mercy, the judge hollered to him, "Just a minute; come back here. I'm curious. Tell me, what does a spotted owl taste like?"

The man thought for a minute and then said, "Judge, the meat tastes a little bit like between a bald eagle and a seagull!"

The lumber crisis in Leavenworth with its spotted owls, however, was met with creative options. The town fathers at the time decided to re-create Leavenworth into a German mountain town. The surrounding majestic mountains cooperate well with this vision. And the *Sound of Music* is dramatized outside in that backdrop during the summer.

Now Leavenworth has the cultural and visual feel of a real German town in the Northwest, and you can even get an authentic, tasty *wienerschnitzel* with *spätzle* noodles, and a *sachertorte* for dessert. And don't forget the German *bier*!

Scheduling the Operation

Once back in Seattle at the U.W. Medical Center, we again checked in and were ushered to Dr. Brant Oelschlager's office. He went over my tests and scans and said he would be glad to do my operation.

The only negative in his mind was the schedule. It would be almost three months before he could schedule my operation. And the reality was the cancer could metastasize during that time, making an operation superfluous.

An oncologist from the hospital joined our discussions and recommended I do some chemo treatments in the meantime. That would ensure the cancer did not get outside the tumor walls. We scheduled the operation date and headed back to Bend.

More Chemo Infusions…Ouch!

In the next consultation with my Bend oncologist, Dr. Martin, three different types of chemo were suggested to solve the potential metastasis issue.

One of those was called Herceptin. As a result of my third endoscopy just prior to this, it was discovered that my cells had morphed from their original form into HER-2 cells. Often this is the type of cell found in breast cancer, and Herceptin is very effective in knocking out the HER-2 cells in those patients.

So Dr. Martin wanted me to take Herceptin and along with it take two other chemo drugs: Oxiplaten and Xeloda.

The first two could be infused through the veins. Xeloda, however, was a two-day pump issue, and therefore, Dr. Martin wanted to install a port in my chest.

Because I was only having chemo for a couple months, I didn't want a port. (Even though a port is a great way to take infusions or give blood tests for longer periods of time. Sheri had a port for a couple years without problems and had it flushed every six weeks.)

So I asked if there was any other way to do the chemo besides a port? Dr. Martin then said I could take Xeloda in the form of tablets. A regimen would be six tablets per day for twelve days. This would be repeated every three weeks until a month before my operation. This was ideal for me for several reasons, one being a trip we had planned to Arizona.

(*Lesson*: It pays to discuss your issues with the doctor and ask questions. If I hadn't in this case, a port would have been surgically put in, and I never would have known another option existed!)

When my first chemo treatment came, I headed for the St. Charles Cancer Center for my infusion. I found the Herceptin to be an easy chemo to tolerate.

The other one I had infused at the same time, the FU-LF-Oxiplaten, had terrible side effects. That toxin hit my nervous system quite hard after the first two-hour infusion.

By mid-afternoon of that day my fingers were numb when I touched something cold. And "cold" was the order of the day! This was winter in Oregon, and every door handle was COLD! Ouch! I actually put on a glove or grabbed a cloth just to open the door.

In addition to this side effect, I also had fatigue and nausea, which are common effects of chemo.

Fortunately, I saw Dr. Martin again before my second round of chemo, so I begged off on the Oxiplaten. By this time my fingers were almost back to normal and gloves no longer needed.

Because no studies proved Oxiplaten was essential for my case, which was already outside the norm, Dr. Martin agreed to stop this chemo. I continued with the Herceptin infusions and Xeloda tablets.

(*Lesson*: Again, this shows we should be responsible for our own treatment, and doctors are receptive to much of our desires and needs if in their judgment it will not affect us adversely.)

So this was my protocol two more times as I patiently waited for my esophagectomy. I must also say, however, that I tried to put the operation out of my mind. I definitely was not looking forward to it as the days passed by and operation day approached.

Back to Seattle for the Final Time!

The days on the calendar clicked off and finally it was March 8, 2017, our day to drive to Seattle. We discovered a sweet, two-bedroom cottage for rent through Air B&B,[45] only one mile away from the hospital.

We booked it when we saw it online, and upon arrival in Seattle, we unpacked and settled in. It had everything we needed, except a TV. That was a little disappointing to me since I'm a "news junkie." But the withdrawal from the high blood pressure CNN or FOX creates was good for my system!

March 9 was a big day. In the morning I had my PET scan to ensure no metastasis had occurred. Then I had a blood panel test to ensure I was fit for the operation. In the afternoon I had my final consultation with Dr. Oelschlager.

The tests and time flew by, and mid-afternoon we were ushered into Dr. Oelschlager's office. He came in with an assistant and informed me the cancer had NOT metastasized. So we were good to go with the operation in five days.

I received more instructions and asked my questions before he left. The next time I would see him would be on Tuesday, March 16—Operation Day.

Time to Kill the Twenty Cancer Soldiers!

Again, the intervening days ticked away. They were enjoyable. We saw some Seattle friends, and on Monday, March 13, I had my final meal—a steak dinner at the Ram

---

[45] https://www.airbnb.com/.

Brewery and Restaurant in the College Mall near the cottage.

The closer I came to the deadline, the more nervous I was. Second guessing my decision was a reality. Did I make the right decision to have the operation? What if it didn't go well? How would I come out of this? What am I going to have to live with as a result?

But the illustration of the twenty soldiers was always in my mind as a counter-weight. Good alternatives didn't exist. And our conscious step-by-step processing made this a solid decision.

So…into the battle I went—or actually Dr. Oelschlager and his team were going into battle in my behalf, and the prayers of many were ahead of all of us.

O-Day came on March 14, 2017, and Sheri delivered me to the hospital in my sweats. Check-in went fast, and we walked over to the section of the hospital where the operation would be done.

My room was designated, and I went in to strip and put on the clean, beautiful, white robe with the tie strings in back I'm never able to tie shut.

From that point on the room was filled with very capable doctors, interns, and nurses, coming and going for one reason or another known only to them, but also shared with me.

My IV was hooked up, my vitals were taken, and a statement giving permission to use my tumor tissue for research was signed. I was surely glad to do that so the tumor could be good for something instead of good for nothing.

My First Medical Decision That Day

Suddenly two pain control docs arrived and let me know they were there to insert an epidural into my lower back by the spine. They listed off the potential side effects I could have with this method, and my ears perked up when they said, "There's a slight chance you could also be paralyzed from the waist down!"

This took me by surprise. What is it about medicine and medical procedures? Again, in my mind, the solution was almost worse than the problem. It's like the medicine advertised on TV that solves the problem of coughing but could end up giving you lymphoma cancer.

And I wasn't sure I wanted someone sticking needles into my spinal sack to control the pain and end up in a wheelchair. The operation I was facing was trouble enough.

So I asked what options I had.

They informed me I only had two options. The other option besides the epidural was to have pain meds administered through my IV line. These two sharp young docs did inform me, however, that the IV route was not as effective as blocking the pain with an epidural.

But again, they said, "This is your decision." That made matters worse. Who wants to decide to potentially end up in a wheelchair?

So my mind started into overdrive processing my choices. Finally, considering all the prayers sent upstairs on my behalf, and knowing God's will was the ultimate backdrop to my life, I told them to go ahead with the epidural.

I leaned forward and they plugged in the needle. Then they fixed the position of the needle with tape. I felt nothing, laid back, and waited to be wheeled into the operating room.

Before the aide came to move me out, Dr. Oelschlager showed up to calm my nerves, inform me he didn't drink coffee when I suggested he get a cup, and said the operation would take about six hours.

As I reflected on the "coffee issue" and the number of times Dr. Oelschlager had done this operation in the past twenty years, I realized his hands would be very steady, to my benefit.

He left my room, the aide came into it, and I was wheeled down the hall to another section of the hospital for Operation Day.

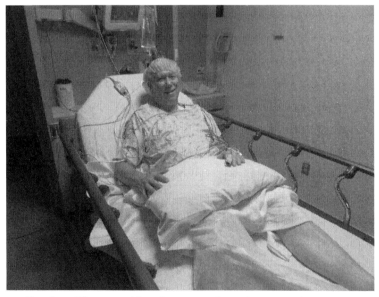

Ready with my epidural to move into the operating room.

Waking Up, and Glad I Did!

From this point on something must have been going through the IV to deaden my memory because I remember nothing of what happened next...except that I woke up in my Intensive Care Unit room late in the afternoon.

I had no pain since the pain block was working well. Sheri and our three daughters were there to greet me, groggy as I was. Again I don't remember much of that first night in the ICU but obviously made it through, or you wouldn't be reading this.

The next day I was wheeled to another section of the hospital and into my recovery room, glad the recovery process was going more, rather than less, normal. Or going better than worse.

How Do You Like Tubes?

My recovery room became my "everything" for the next five days. The fact is the room was full of tubes. Here's the Dr. Seuss-style poem I created regarding this reality. What else do you do in a recovery room besides play poet?

I think we could call the title of this ditty "Tubing!"

Tubes are up. Tubes are down.
Making me a little clown!
Tubes are here. Tubes are there.
Those crazy Tubes are everywhere!

My IV was hooked up to a tube ending in a bag of liquid perched high above my head. Its purpose was to keep me hydrated.

Another tube, connected to my IV, ended in a bag of liquid painkiller, also stationed above my head. Its purpose was to give a shot of anesthetic to my upper chest whenever I needed it. At least I had control of that button and could press it when I wanted pain relief.

I had a tube coming upwards from my stomach through my nose and hooked to a sucking machine. Its purpose was to keep my stomach acid controlled. Now without a hiatal valve, I had nothing to stop the acid from pushing up into my throat—not a good result with an anastomosis.

Then through a stomach area hole entering my intestine, I had my feeding tube. The tube was taped to my skin and hooked up to a pump that kept me fed with liquid nutrition, similar to Ensure. No taste involved, but a lot of sustenance and noise.

This feeding was essential since nothing could go down my new "stomach esophagus" until day three after the operation. Then I would be able to eat only a clear-liquid diet for a couple days, proceeding to soft foods like yogurt.

Since it would be weeks until I was eating enough food through my mouth and could rid myself of this tube, it was my constant partner—actually keeping me alive.

The final nail in my tube coffin was the cord to the shin massager.

One side effect of lying in bed for twenty-three hours a day was the potential for blood clots in the legs. To offset these potential clots, a shin massager was wrapped around each leg and would inflate and deflate as long as connected to electricity. Since these cords were short, my recovery room mobility was even more severely limited.

Recovery Days...and Terrifying Nights

During the daytime, off and on interns and docs stopped by. There was never a dull moment. Nurses were regularly busy doing all of their tasks related to me — waking, poking, prodding, changing my position, etc. You know the drill.

The TV was on the stations I enjoyed (back to the news). And even though it was Seattle, known for its rain, I had some sunny days with rays beaming through my hospital window cheering me up.

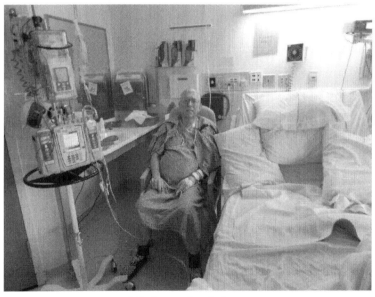

My home for 5 days

The nights, however, were terrible. The line between day and night was blurred. Because I would sleep intermittently during the day, it was difficult to fall asleep at a normal bedtime.

And sleeping was a chore in itself. I had at least five pillows on my bed, maneuvered for comfort. The only position allowing sleep was a halfway sitting position. And with the tubes coming at me from every direction, tying me up, my ability to peacefully find a good sleeping position was difficult.

So I found myself watching TV until after midnight, trying to get to sleep. The longer this situation went on, the more anxious I got. One night I'd doze off at 1am. The next would be 2am. Then the nurse would show up at 5am for a checkup and a blood pressure reading, waking me from a deep sleep.

Often, I would also slide down on the bed and need help to get back up into a comfortable sleep-sitting position. This couldn't be done without help, so I'd push the red button to call a nurse in to help me shuttle back up.

After several nights of this routine, I was embarrassed to call the nurse again. So I decided to try shifting positions on my own. To my chagrin, some of the tubes got tangled with each other like a noose around my body.

To solve this, I disconnected the shin machine, only to find those cords tangled around my legs. This put me in a such an awkward position from other tubes, I couldn't reach them to gain freedom.

Finally, in desperation I hit the red button and called in the marines. She was masquerading as my night nurse and got me resettled where I wanted to be in the first place. But this all happened with a gentle rebuke to call her the next time I wanted to shift positions.

As she wisely indicated, my physical condition was in such a fragile state yet, they didn't want anything to upset the "tube cart."

Live and learn. It's hard to teach a new trick to an old dog who's been self-sufficient most of his life and hasn't wrestled with a bunch of tubes!

Recovery Going Better Than Expected

With the encouragement of Sheri, my daughters, the nursing staff, and docs, my attitude and efforts were paying off in recovery.

Blood tests were indicating good health. My vitals were good. My scars and arthroscopic chest holes were healing well. My body had no pain so I didn't need to push the little red opioid button. (I did push it two times during my stay to use the painkiller as a sleep aid—I did sleep then.)

He Who Walks…Heals!

The first day in the ICU unit, the nurse told me, "He who walks, heals." One of my daily routines was to walk a mile around the hospital floor. I took this to heart and met my quota each day, starting out quite slow, but picking up speed as the days clicked by.

Actually, the walk with Sheri around the recovery unit was an enjoyable and anticipated break from simply lying in bed for twenty-four hours.

Of course, I had to drag my IV pole with me, but the interlude was a delightful change from the four white walls of my hospital room. When walking I could enjoy the white walls of the hallway!

By three days after the operation, my whiskers were getting long. Sheri came with an electric razor, and I started feeling more normal again once the fuzz was gone. A shampoo at the room sink and a wash of the upper body made my day. I was feeling like a million bucks!

On day five after the operation a nurse came and helped me with a full body wash, and I was starting to think I could soon leave the hospital.

Night five was another bad one for me. Anxiety. Lack of sleep. Some claustrophobia from tube constriction. Wishes for daylight to come soon. Attempts to get the mind off the whole situation so I could sink into sleep.

So when day six arrived and the intern team came in to assess me at 7:00 in the morning, I asked, "Could I get out of here by tonight? I really don't want to spend another night in this bed. I'd rather be in our cottage under the care of my wife if everything can be cleared for that to happen."

The head intern replied, "We'll see what we can do." An hour later another intern stopped by to say they were going to try and get me out by the evening. Great! My spirits revived. With those words, the eclipse felt like it was entirely over.

That kicked everything into high gear, including my attitude. Here's what I had to accomplish to get out of Floor 4 of the hospital and into my cottage bed:

- Another full body wash by myself
- Vitals in top condition
- Bowel movement
- Catheter removed
- Emptying of the bladder with a certain amount of liquid
- The epidural removed and pain monitored
- Mobility judged and a mile walk taken
- Feeding tube disconnected
- Lesson by the nutritionist on how to use a portable feeding tube pump and liquid food

- Kiss my wife while standing—not necessary but surely desired by me

Will the Throat Connection Hold?

But first I had to pass the BIG hurdle. I needed a barium test to determine if the throat connection (anastomosis) was sutured and healed well enough so no leakage would result.

In hindsight I realized this was a major part of the operation and an essential recovery element. Fortunately for me, Dr. Oelschlager's percentage of leakage was only 1%.

If I was in the 1%, however, and some saliva would slip through the suture, a medical patch-up would be needed. This meant spending more days in the hospital for the repair. Obviously, this is not what I had in mind for my life. But some things in life we simply can't control even if we want to.

I waited patiently for the trip to the barium x-ray room. Finally, the aide showed up with a wheelchair to hustle me off to the barium picture lab in the lower sanctums of this huge hospital.

We pulled into the area with a screeching halt of the wheelchair. A cheerful nurse administered the barium through a straw from a bottle and stood me up on an x-ray machine. Two doctors administered the test and analyzed results through a couple monitors.

Shortly after that, one came out of the monitoring room and said, "The barium seems to be stalled in your stomach and isn't moving into your intestine. We want you to sit up in your wheelchair for ten minutes and see if that moves it forward."

I sat there as the minutes ticked by with my fingers crossed, prayers expressed, and some shuffle movement of my lower body. I figured if I bounced slightly up or down, it might help the barium move. Was that cheating? I didn't know, but I surely wanted a positive verdict after those ten minutes slipped past.

Finally, the nurse helped me shuffle on to the standing platform again for another x-ray.

Through the window of the analysis room filled with the monitors, I saw the two doctors in expressive conversation. Oh, oh! Was the anastomosis sealed? Did the barium enter my intestine? What would I be facing now? They surely looked animated with concern!

At last the doctors came back to me and one said, "Are you up for some good news?"

That was a "duh" question. Of course, my answer to that question was a hearty "yes," and I was hoping he wouldn't follow by asking, "Now do you want the bad news?"

He said, "There is NO leakage, and the barium has entered your intestine. It was probably stalled because of the inflammation of that area from the operation. We see no problems. You have a green light to proceed!"

I was one happy former esophageal cancer patient. I didn't realize at the time of the operation that it would be the anastomosis which was the critical issue. If that aspect was not done properly in the operation, much more hassle would hit my life.

Now however, with a tight and successful anastomosis, my recovery was moving ahead at a solid pace! More cause for joy! More sunshine returning to my life.

The aide wheeled me back to my room at a fast pace, with another item on the checklist accomplished so I could get out of there. We screeched to another halt, this time in my recovery room. I disembarked to check off the remainder of those items as the day progressed.

Each item on the list was accomplished in its timing and way. The final consultation was with the feeding tube nurse who informed me how to input the liquid from a can into the machine and set it at a proper feeding speed. I looked at a couple cans but didn't see any of them labeled as "steak."

Wonderful Release!

At 7:00 p.m. the evening of my sixth day in the hospital, one of the interns came to my room and said I could be released into the loving hands and care of my wife!

The release paperwork was completed. My meager belongings in the room were quickly packed into a bag. I put on my sweats and shoes and hustled out of the hospital down into the bowels of the parking garage. Sheri revved up the car, and on we went to the cottage for my post-operative recovery!

8
WHAT HAPPENS WHEN THE DOC SAYS "GOODBYE?"

I already mentioned our cozy cottage one mile from the hospital. Dr. Oelschlager wanted me to stay close by the hospital after release for at least nine days in case any complications arose. This cottage was ideal for us.

Recovery at the Cottage

Located in a quiet Seattle neighborhood with sidewalks, I could get my daily exercise without a lot of stress. Having no TV meant I could peacefully read and sleep without that temptation. I did a lot of sleeping as my body used my limited energy to heal.

Regarding exercise, Sheri and I are still actively walking at least one mile several days a week. Most cancer docs recommend this strategy as a healthy way to hold cancer back.

Someone said, "Listen to your body and do what it tells you." Even though I'm more cerebral than subjective, that adage was wisdom for me. When the body said, "I'm tired," I took a nap. When the body indicated, "You have some energy to use," I took a walk. I ate the prescribed liquid and soft foods several times a day as well as kept my feeding pump going with the cans of nutrition.

By the way, I found out Medicare does not cover the feeding pump and canned nutrition costs, so the quicker we can get off these the more money we save out of our own pockets.

All the Complicated Sleep Factors

Sleeping was a unique challenge. Prior to the operation I went on Amazon and found a full length, foam mattress for $69.00. It was twin bed size so we cut it down to a ½ queen bed size and planned to use it on our queen bed at home.

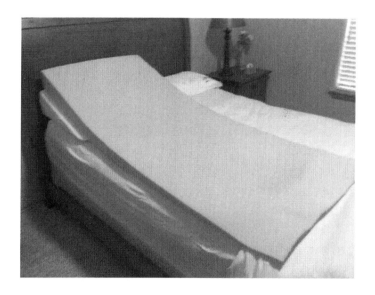

We took this along to Seattle and had it ready for me to use on the queen bed at the cottage.

An hour into the first night at the cottage, however, we realized Sheri would not sleep well with my breathing noise and fussing around as I tried to get comfortable many times during the night.

My body also indicated I should have something more upright than the foam with a couple pillows on it for my head. The closer I slept to a "normal" sleep position, the more pressure I found on my throat. I needed to relieve that through a more upright position and give it time to heal.

Sleeping in a more angled upright position also helped control acid reflux. While the reflux would most likely not cause another tumor in my stomach tube as it did in my esophagus, I now had no hiatal valve to hold back the acid. Gravity is the survivor's best friend, but in order for that to be effective, an esophageal cancer survivor must sleep on an incline.

Fortunately, the cottage had two bedrooms. We decided to set up the second one for me and let Sheri sleep in her normal way in the first bedroom.

To gain the upright position I needed, we found an old lawn chair in the backyard that could be manipulated to put my feet and back up and down.

It was ideal for what I needed immediately after being released from the hospital. It took the pressure off the operation points and gave relief to the tightness of the throat.

Initially I slept in that chair for a full night's sleep. After several nights passed, however, I would switch between the chair and the foam mattress laid out on the single bed. A couple pillows on the foam with an additional short "incline pillow" gave me more angle for throat stricture and acid reflux control.

This pattern for night sleeping allowed my healing to continue with a little variety, and I gained strength day by day. (Notice my blow-up neck pillow. I still sleep with a neck pillow since it puts my head at a good angle for sleeping and control of snoring.)

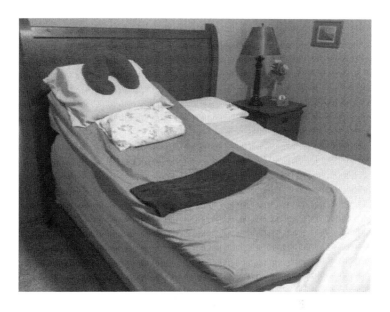

How to Gain Excellent Sleep at Home

Elevate!

At home, I started with an incline of a 4-inch rise of the mattress itself by putting boards on the frame under the mattress. Then I have another 4-inch incline because of the full-length foam mattress I mentioned.

In addition, to get even more height, I added another shorter "wedge" pillow purchased from Bed, Bath and Beyond.

Finally, on top of all this, I sleep with a neck pillow on my normal pillow. This 12-14-inch incline helps stabilize my body to sleep on my back all night, and it didn't cost very much. It also has somehow controlled my tendency to snore, at least periodically. (I'm sure loss of weight helped with the snoring issue as well.)

Keep from Sliding Down.

One other issue to mention: when sleeping on an incline the body's natural tendency is to slide downward during the night.

In the dead of night, I often found my feet hitting the end board, and because I was now lower on the incline, the acid would kick up into my throat, waking me and making me go for some water!

To solve that issue, initially I rolled up a towel and put it under the sheet at the foot end of the bed. This worked okay and kept me from sliding down most of the time.

However, an even better method I discovered is to fold a bath towel in quarters and place this just below the buttocks under the legs. The material itself doesn't slide easily and therefore holds me in place better than a rolled towel at my feet, which was also a little uncomfortable.

This setup went well for the first six months of recovery after the operation and controlled acid reflux most nights unless my body still slid down and got too level. Then the horrid acid taste would wake me for some water to dissipate the discomfort.

I now have a lot of respect for the toughness of the internal stomach tissues. It handles this very strong acid on a constant 24/7 basis! Wow, what an organ.

Get a Good Bed!

Since this sleep condition will follow me all the days of my remaining life, Sheri and I finally decided to bite the cost bullet and replace our queen bed, loaded with various foam pads and pillows. This was replaced with a king bed that automatically elevates by the touch of a key pad.

We found one at the Mattress Firm Labor Day Sale and are paying for it monthly at 0% interest. This means we pay the frame/mattress cost off over the next few years at only $59.00 per month. That's not too aggravating on the pocketbook for ensuring an ongoing, good night's sleep.

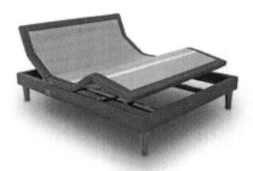

Our frame elevates in three locations: on the foot end, the back-incline area, and the head end. It also has a nightlight and built in massager to help loosen and move the lymph system.

Now we each sleep on our own twin bed and mattress allowing each of us to determine our own comfort angle for the night. Since this bed has a "leg lift" function, sliding down is not the major problem it once was although I still use a folded towel to hold me up as well. My neck pillow still keeps my throat at a good angle and head elevated.

All of that provides a very good night's sleep...on my back.

Sleeping on My Back

Sleep studies indicate there are at least four stages to a good night's sleep. The first two stages bring us toward the needed sleep stages, "delta" and "REM". REM stands for "rapid eye movement" and is the deep and desired stage of nightly sleep. According to the research, we cycle through these stages about every ninety minutes per night.[46]

However, each time we turn over on our side or disrupt our sleeping pattern in some way, our bodies are kicked back into the early stages. If we toss and turn too much in a night, we never hit the last two stages of deep and needed sleep.

That's why sleeping on our backs is the best type of sleep—no side movement back and forth to disrupt our sleep stages!

I had to retrain my body to rest this way since I was a stomach and side sleeper. Now I enjoy this style of sleeping and have slept well since my operation. The neck pillow was important in this retraining since it kept me "fixed" and unable to get on my side.

Another positive side effect of the back-sleeping position is no more of the restless-leg syndrome which once plagued me.

---

[46] American Sleep Apnea Association, (https://www.sleephealth.org/sleep-health/importance-of-sleep-understanding-sleep-stages/).

The Complicated Feeding Tube Factors

Flushing the Feeding Tube!

One night-issue I faced at the cottage immediately, and then at home later, was the feeding tube. It was necessary to flush the tube about every four hours to keep it from blocking.

This meant a couple times each night I'd make a short trip to the kitchen to disconnect the stomach feeding tube, push some water through the tube with a push tool, and reinsert the pump hose into the stomach connection.

This was no major issue except it disrupted sleep a couple times each night.

We were about six days into cottage recovery time when once I waited too long to flush my stomach feeding tube. The next time I flushed it, no water would push through because the tube was totally blocked. It felt like I hit a cement wall. My liquid stomach eating, therefore, ground to a solid halt.

This happened on a Saturday, of course, as most emergencies do, but we dutifully got in the car and headed for the hospital, hoping to solve this problem.

The nurse and doc on duty tried flushing with no success. So meat tenderizer was ordered from the pharmacy for the problem. (We found out that Coca Cola works just as well—and to think we normally drink Coke as a soft drink! It's actually a gut tenderizer? Ugh.

While we waited for the tenderizer, the doc tried loosening the blockage with a small wire. Then Sheri took the plastic flushing tool and did a push-pull, plunger type motion a number of times. This loosened the stuck food in the tube, the blockage cleared, and we were back to normal operations.

From then on I was very conscientious to keep that tube clean and did the procedure religiously every four hours.

All the "Home Sweet Home" Factors

Post-Operative Consultation

After nine days of managing my recovery at the cottage, we had our post-operative consultation with one of the interns. Dr. Oelschlager had delegated this task to one of his team.

After checking my vitals one last time and sharing with the intern how I was feeling and doing nine days out from my surgery, we met with the nutritionist.

Her task was to get me off the feeding tube while maintaining a certain healthy level of weight for five or six days.

This appointment started at 9:00 a.m., and we were done with everything at 11:00 a.m. I was feeling great, buoyed by a good night's sleep, by the energy created from the liquid food diet, and by the adrenalin pumped into my body because of a good consultation and my release from Seattle!

Was This a Wise Decision?

Feeling great in the moment, I was eager to get moving. So on the way to the car, I said to Sheri, "How about if we go back to the cottage, pack up, and drive the six hours back to Bend today?"

Since we had been gone from home for three weeks, she liked that idea as well. So two hours later we left the cottage in good condition, said goodbye to our friendly neighbors, loaded the car, and took off for Bend, Oregon. I was feeling so good I even drove a couple hours on the route home.

How wonderful it was to open the garage, go into a cold house, start the furnace, and know we were finally home!

The date was March 30, 2017. We had been gone twenty-two days.

Pushing Too Hard!

When I woke up the next day to enjoy our first day back home, I was a total mess. Tired. Hurting. Anxious. The six-hour trip home, piled on the two hours of energy spent on the packing, piled on the two hours at the hospital for the post-op, had taken a heavy toll on me.

It took me a week to recover from that "exuberant mistake" and get back to the condition I was in before we got into the car for the drive home.

In 20/20 hindsight I learned "feeling good" does not translate into body strength and energy after such a traumatic operation. This is a time I should have turned "macho" into "wuss."

The better plan would have been to go back to the cottage, relax for a time, take a leisure walk, pack later in the day, and then leave for Bend the next day—as was our original plan. Oh well. Live and learn! But at least I was nursing my mistake at home!

Entering Back into the Mainstream of Life

Back in Bend we had many friends concerned for us. They followed my cancer journey, prayed for us, sent words of encouragement, and were very glad to have us back home safe, sound, and in decent shape.

So they wanted to visit. I discovered I only had energy for one two-hour visit a day for the first three weeks back. At the hospital, one of my nurses informed me I would have a limited energy bank, and I could expend it too quickly.

That advice proved to be very true. The body needed most of my energy for healing, and guest visits took much energy as well, especially for an introvert.

So as much as we wanted friends to stop by, we had to limit that activity for several weeks. Often during those first three weeks, after a visit I would take a two-hour nap to replenish my energy bank.

Going out of the house also tapped into my energy bank account. I normally let Sheri drive to save my energy, and then I'd push the cart around the grocery store to get some exercise. Even though this activity was not too strenuous, upon arriving home I would often need another nap.

Normally I got my planned exercise with a daily neighborhood walk after napping, when my energy was replenished and I was emotionally up for going outside.

My energy bank account got larger and larger as the weeks rolled by and my body healed more and more. After six weeks I felt my energy was almost back to normal. Daily naps were done, and I could operate on my normal schedule as I had before the operation. That has been true up to today.

The 'What to Eat' or 'What Not to Eat' Factors

I wondered how food would go after I had the operation. Would I be able to swallow okay? Would I be able to eat anything? Could I have my favorite foods again or not? Could I drink a good beer with a pizza? (Bend, Oregon, has thirty-two micro-breweries and some great-tasting craft beer.)

Basically, I've had no mechanical issue with eating again after my operation. Swallowing goes normal.

My first issue was weaning myself off the feeding tube, with its cans of nourishment, while making up the difference by eating real food through my new stomach digestive system.

I was on the feeding tube for about one month before that weaning process was complete and I could have my stomach feeding tube removed. Because of the type of feeding tube I had, it came out in a simple five-minute procedure.

My second issue with food is a lingering one I'm still managing today—to know how much to eat at one time and what types of foods my new system will handle well.

My body pushes me toward vegetarian type foods and away from beef and pork, which are harder for my new system to digest.

Soups always look good and digest well. And having various salads in the fridge is an easy way to ensure I eat more than three times a day. For me that variety of salads includes potato, pasta, three bean, pea and cheese, coleslaw, and feta-olive.[47]

Chicken and fish digest well, and that's the issue: what can the newly formed stomach digest easily without benefit of the enzymes of the removed esophagus?

Also, an easier digestion process is created by excessive chewing. If repeated chewing occurs, a good amount of saliva enzyme is put into the food prior to swallowing. With no enzymatic action from the now absent esophagus, only the stomach takes on the big digestive job. If the food

---

[47] According to the Mayo Clinic it takes 6 to 8 hours for food to pass through the stomach and small intestine. Digestibility refers to how much of a food can be broken down into necessary nutrients used by the body. It normally takes up to 24-72 hours to digest red meat, depending on your digestive tract, (https://www.mayoclinic.org/digestive-system/expert-answers/faq-20058340).

is chewed well, that process is much easier for the stomach.

Usually within 45-60 minutes after I eat something, I know if the digestion of the food went well (seamless without thought), or if I'll have a sick feeling in my stomach for a short period of time.

I've fought off the dry-heaves a few times, but mostly it's either a short nausea period, causing me to think about the food I just ate, or the food moves well through the system and I never give it another thought. (As of this writing, I very rarely think about food anymore—only about when to eat.)

The further away from the operation I get and the more the body heals, the more foods I can eat with better appetite. After eight months, I'm enjoying ground beef again, but steak still seems a stretch because of its solid consistency and the difficulty to break the meat down through chewing. But now I'm confident I will get around to a nice juicy T-bone at some point in the near future—maybe on January 6, 2018?

After the operation, the nutritionist recommended I eat smaller portions of food at least five times a day rather than three larger meals. This is often difficult, depending on where I'm at during the day and what I'm doing. Being away from home or traveling presents additional issues.

I hate the fact that food is such a focus of my day, and weight loss is a continual concern. I've lost thirty-five pounds since the operation, but fortunately I had some extra weight to lose. After eight months on the downward trend, the scales show my body finally balanced out at 165 pounds. This is a very healthy weight for me, but one I haven't been at since high school. (Ouch! That's over 50 years!)

The big concern with weight loss is my BMI (body mass index) factor. My nutritionist put this factor in my mind, and initially I was probably too consumed with it. The concern was that too much weight loss meant the body was self-consuming muscle instead of fat. The BMI tracks the muscle mass.

My daughter, who's a nurse, said I have nothing to worry about. I was 198 pounds when I went in for the operation. After six months I was 168 pounds. Now I'm 165. A normal BMI for my height is 18.5 to 24. At 168 pounds I have a BMI of 22. So I could slip in weight all the way to 130 pounds without concern to get to the low end of normal at 18.5. (You can find BMI calculators through Google.)

At this point as I track my progress, I'm confident I'll get beyond these food issues. At seven months out from the operation, this is getting better for me by the month. My appetite is good, and most foods look good. Digestion is going basically well. What more could I ask?

Where will I be on this issue at one year or more out? Time will tell. However, if the cancer is gone, as I believe it is, and managing the food issue is the only disability I have from the operation, I will consider this on the positive side of my experience!

Is the Cancer Gone?

Dr. Castillo in Mexico warned me, "Dave, cancer is never gone. So stay on the natural therapies."

This is good advice from a cancer doctor of thirty years' experience. Although I'm not taking all my former supplements eight months out from the operation, we are having our <blueberry, kale, whey powder, orange juice> smoothie five mornings a week and a <carrot, apple, onion,

ginger root, turmeric root, radish, beet juice, garlic clove> juice five afternoons per week.

Unless there is a hidden cancer cell, or even one that might develop again down the road, there is no indication on the radar screen that cancer is still in my body.

During the operation, Dr. Oelschlager tested a two-inch margin in the stomach and a three-inch margin in the chest. No cancer cells presented themselves in the concurrent pathology tests.

He removed seventeen lymph nodes that were then tested during the operation. None of those showed any cancer.

And the tumor itself was still contained in my esophagus with the five outer layers of the esophagus regenerating.

Therefore, is the cancer gone? Yes, in terms of all visible measurements and a 50% survival rate. No, in terms of allopathic and naturopathic best practice and experience and a 50% survival rate.

Again, which side of the equation will I end up experiencing? (And the God-thing is a major positive in the equation as well. See the next three chapters on that subject.)

As I said before, I started out with Stage-II, T3 N1 MX as my diagnosis. The operation uncovered the fact my condition was more like Stage-I, T1 N0 M0 just before my operation.

This had to be the result of a combination of the following factors:
1) the natural healing powers of the body,
2) chemo and radiation to knock it back,
3) naturopathic treatments, and
4) the healing hand of God (Jehovah Rapha).

So for me the twenty soldiers have been defeated. If five more show up, we'll deal with that through new cancer treatments discovered after this time; perhaps through chemo designed to knock it back or through natural means again!

No other options exist—except one for those of us who believe in Jesus as a healer, and that's "divine healing"—the supernatural touch of God on a person's sickness to eliminate it today. And in Chapters 9-12 of this book I discuss various aspects of this twenty-first century reality as a possibility for our health situation.

9

IS THERE A HEALER TODAY BY THE NAME OF JESUS?

Probably most of us recognize some spiritual aspect to our existence, however we describe that or however we worship—if we do.

This is no exception for me. When I first learned I had cancer, the spiritual aspects of my cancer journey were uppermost in my mind. These spiritual beliefs had a significant impact on my health journey and contributed to my health outcomes.

I said earlier I would include my thoughts on the spiritual aspects of healing. So this chapter and the next three cover this important aspect of my cancer eclipse story including, in Chapter 12, my responses to some questions others raised about my cancer eclipse.

Because this is so real to me and was the foundation upon which my cancer battles were fought, I'm not pulling any punches in these chapters.

I'm telling my spiritual story as I see it through my glasses. At the same time, I realize my glasses don't define the standard upon which reality and truth are measured.

So if you want to discuss any part of what I'm sharing, I'd be very happy to hear from you. I'm still on a learning curve in life and know I have something to learn from you if we do connect. Write me: CancerEclipse@gmail.com

My Basic Spiritual Premise

Each of us probably has a definition of what we consider spiritual. And there are many and various "spiritualities" in our world today. Therefore, at the outset I'd like to define my view of spirituality so you know my angle in approaching this subject.

First of all, you probably realize from the title of this chapter, I'm a believer in Jesus Christ and identify as one of His disciples today. But I would classify myself as one of His weak disciples based on the issues I've wrestled with over the years and the things I've done, of which I'm not proud.

Yet the God of the Bible is Love, and Jesus came to reveal that fact to us. He offers forgiveness, love, and help no matter who we are or what we face, which includes sickness.

I'm encouraged by the fact that those following Jesus 2,000 years ago also had their human weaknesses and shortcomings. Jesus accepted and loved them; so I know He can do that with me as well.

Secondly, I also believe Jesus is God, who entered this world in a human body and proved that fact by His powerful resurrection from the grave. Did He actually rise from the dead?

That question has been debated, and most world religions have some "take" on this event. Which "take" is closer to the truth than the others seems to be the question?

It's interesting to me that in the past 2,000 years of world history with all its very great thinkers, no one has ever disproven the resurrection. Yet there have been many attempts to prove this incident never happened.

In fact, based on the historical documents we have, the evidence seems to point to a resurrection rather than some other view of that event, like the swoon theory.

In my view, the resurrection is the key element of Jesus' life. It's on this recorded happening the case for Jesus either succeeds or fails.

If He did not rise from the dead after being crucified and buried as He and others claimed, He is nothing but a hoax. Then all who follow Him are deceived fools, including me.

[Note: There are only four basic opinions one can hold about the identity of Jesus that make any logical sense. So if we have an opinion about Him, it falls into one of these four views. I've described these views in Appendix F: What is Your Present Opinion of Jesus?]

How I "Met" Jesus as a Living Person

It was in 1962 when I actually "met" Jesus as a living person and committed my life to Him as my Lord. Of course, this was not a meeting with Him in the flesh since He left Earth 2,000 years ago.

Rather Jesus now operates in a different dimension, outside our four human dimensions. My encounter with Him happened in the spiritual realm, so it was a spiritual experience.

My spiritual awakening occurred one night at Hope College in Holland, Michigan. Alone in my dorm room, I consciously realized a soul-altering fact: Basically, I was a rebel against God because I wanted to live my life on my terms, in my way. I did not want His input in my life on any level.

At the same time, I knew I was a lawbreaker of God's law, summarized in the Ten Commandments.[48] According to the Bible, these two realities of my life created a relational and spiritual separation between God and me. Unless something was done about those realities, this separation would last for eternity.

When I started understanding the essence of all this, it felt to me like I was stuck with an "eternal death sentence" and had to act in order to change my spiritual condition and situation. He took His step toward me when Jesus came. Now it was my turn to take a step toward Him.

Today I can't exactly express all my thoughts that night in 1962 in my dorm room. (That's a long time ago, and "half-heimers" doesn't help).

My thoughts centered on this stream of consciousness: "How is it working for me to run life on my own, doing what I want every moment? I'm totally treating people selfishly and disregarding my Creator."

---

[48] The Ten Commandments are listed in Exodus 20:1-17. I have summarized them here:

(1) God must be and remain supreme in our lives.

(2) We must not make or worship any idol.

(3) We must not misuse God's name in any way.

(4) We must keep the Sabbath day holy.

(5) We must honor our father and mother.

(6) We must not murder.

(7) We must not commit adultery.

(8) We must not steal.

(9) We must not testify falsely against our neighbor.

(10) We must not covet what our neighbor has.

Although I was only eighteen years old at the time, I knew deep inside running my life as I thought best was not working too well. And the "death penalty" feeling I had scared me.

Of course, I could blame my religious upbringing for these thoughts and feelings and discount them. But what if there was a God revealed in Jesus? That would certainly change the equation from legend to reality or negatives to positives.

Did I really want to live isolated from God, with no relationship with Him that would take me into eternity? What a lonely place to be.

Because of all the times my parents dragged me to church as a kid, I knew the Bible taught that Jesus paid the "eternal death penalty" for me on the cross. And I heard that somehow this happened through His blood seeping out from the nail holes when He was crucified.

I also knew from my upbringing that through Jesus there was forgiveness with God for any "rebel" who turned to Him with a desire to change.

How and why any of that has meaning in God's economy, or to us here on Earth, is still much of a mystery to me. But that's what Jesus did according to the Bible. Somehow that makes sense to God even though I can't understand it well and have a hard time explaining it.

But I do know when a person decides there could be some credibility in this "Jesus story" and moves their heart and mind toward God as the One who can deliver them from their present situation, something indescribable and wonderful takes place inside them. It's a spiritual happening. It's a spiritual transaction.

That was and is my experience. That night in 1962 I got on my knees by my bed in a small dorm room at college. In that position, for the first time in my life I talked to God from deep in my being. Church going and church prayer had been a charade, a part of my cultural experience. This night I was doing business with the living God of heaven and Earth, and I knew the difference.

I asked Him for forgiveness for my rebellious heart and egotism which pushed me in my way to disobey His way. I thanked God for sending Jesus to help me.

In the Bible, Jesus says, "Listen, I stand at the door of your life and knock. If you hear my voice and open the door, I will come in to you, and have a personal relationship with you" (Revelation 3:20).

That's a great picture of what this spiritual transaction is. So that night I did hear his voice in my spirit. I opened my spiritual door by talking to Jesus and asking Him to come into my life and live with me. In whatever words came out that night in the kneeling prayer, I know I acknowledged Him as my Lord. I told Him I would try to obey Him in life as I went forward.

The Aftermath …

At that moment, on my knees in 1962, I carried out this prayer transaction with a living Jesus I couldn't see with my eyes. This heartfelt call from me to Him somehow changed me internally and set a new trajectory for my life—an eternal trajectory.

As I got up off my knees that night, I had a lightness and joy in my soul. And somehow I had a conviction internally that if I walked out in the street and was killed in an auto accident, I would not simply disintegrate into nothingness, but rather would live forever with God.

That was in 1962 when I was eighteen years old. I can say now in 2017, at the ripe old age of seventy-three, that Jesus has been with me all the way of my life's journey.

And His companionship has been there as I've fought through this cancer eclipse of my life. The confidence I'll be with God for eternity is still a constant encouragement and hope in this dark time.

I'm confident when I pass from this earth I'll see Jesus, the risen Lord, and God, the Father, on the other side of the curtain. These are tremendous spiritual benefits to my life.

Good News for Each of Us!

But the good news is, these things are not only for me. If you're reading this and have never "met" Jesus as the living Savior and Lord, I would highly recommend getting more info on Him from the Bible or a believing friend. Or contact me, and we can have a further conversation about these spiritual truths.

Making the decision to go down this road will help someone understand and appropriate Jesus' power and love in their own life, just as it did for me. A decision to follow Jesus will give them the inner (soul) confidence they will live eternally with God. That's because eternal life is wrapped up in Jesus and in a personal relationship with Him.

Let me share one Bible statement summing up what I've just said: "And this is the record, God gave us eternal life. And this life is in His Son. The person who has the Son, has life. The person who has not the Son of God, has not life" (1 John 5:11-12).

Jesus, the King Who Heals Today

But you might ask, "Dave, isn't it a stretch to go from the claim you have a relationship with God through Jesus to the fact that Jesus can heal someone today and is doing that?"

My answer: That's not too much of a stretch when we realize that Jesus, as the Son of God, is also the King of the powerful Kingdom of God.[49]

In addition, His kingdom has a worldview, or shall we say "kingdom view," in which healing fits well. His kingdom also has kingdom values, one of which is health for everyone in the kingdom.

The kingdom view creates the understanding that Jesus heals, and the kingdom values show that health is of the essence of His kingdom.

What is the Kingdom View?

All of us have questions in our minds and hearts that puzzle us, right? Gaining satisfactory answers to these questions is critical to our ability to function in life. Therefore, we try to answer deep questions in a satisfying way for us. And those answers originate in, and are generated out of, our view of life and the world. Thus, from our personal worldview.

My view of the world determines how I think about life, other people, God, reality, eternity, morality, etc. And those beliefs move me in my decision-making on a daily basis.

---

[49] "Together they [the kings of the earth] will go to war against the Lamb, but the Lamb will defeat them because he is Lord of all lords and King of all kings. And his called and chosen and faithful ones will be with him" (Revelation 17:14 NLT).

Who is the Lamb? Here is John the Baptist's testimony: "The next day John saw Jesus coming toward him and said, 'Look, the Lamb of God, who takes away the sin of the world!'" (John 1:29).

For example, if I believe there is no moral restraint in life concerning cheating someone, then I might become a thief, swindler, or scammer in order to make myself rich. And I won't worry about hurting someone in the process, or I'll justify that in some way within my worldview.

However, if I believe cheating is morally wrong, and I have a value of not hurting others, I won't steal, swindle, or scam and will be sensitive to other's needs.

All of these issues are wrapped up in my worldview, which determines my actions.

I must recognize my view of the world has been formed by many influences that create biases: my family and cultural background, religious training, education, formative friends and enemies, good and bad experiences I've had, etc.

This reality makes my belief system quite subjective and most likely wrong in a number of areas. So seeking truth about this world and life is a vital pursuit for anyone. Challenging one's worldview is also necessary in order to keep growing intellectually and spiritually.

What Essential Questions Does a Worldview Answer?

One of the best descriptions of those basic worldview questions we ask comes from an Indian philosopher, Ravi Zacharias.[50] He identifies four vital areas of a worldview and the strategic questions raised in each area.

---

[50] Born in India in 1946, Zacharias immigrated to Canada with his family in 1966. While pursuing a career in business management, his interest in theology grew; subsequently, he pursued this study during his undergraduate education.

Here are those four critical areas and the vital questions arising from each. Do you ever think about these questions and their answers? I surely do.

- Origins. Where did we come from? How did we get here?

- Meaning. What are we here for? What's the purpose of life? What's the purpose of MY life?

- Morality. What is right and wrong in our world? How do we determine right and wrong in principle?

- Destiny. Where are we headed in life? What happens to us when we die?

Regarding the kingdom view, the Bible unfolds an understanding of how Jesus, the Lamb and King, answers the basic questions of these four areas. The kingdom view of origins, meaning, morality, and destiny is revealed in the Old and New Testaments.

He received his Master of Divinity from Trinity International University in Deerfield, Illinois. Zacharias has authored or edited over 25 books including the Gold Medallion winner *Can Man Live Without God* (Word, 1994).

Zacharias has appeared on CNN, Fox, and other international broadcasts. His weekly radio program, "Let My People Think," airs on 2,337 outlets worldwide, his weekday program, "Just Thinking," on 721, and his one-minute "Just a Thought" on 488 outlets.

It Answers the Question, "Where Does Sickness Come from in the World?"

As an example, let's consider the area of morality. One of Jesus' basic teachings about what is wrong in our world is this: another kingdom exists in our world and is immorally, practically, and powerfully working against the King and the values of His kingdom.

That other kingdom is aptly identified in the Bible as the kingdom of darkness,[51] the kingdom of this world,[52] and the kingdom of Satan,[53] the archenemy of God.

Out of Satan's kingdom, and humanity's fallen nature, comes all that is wrong with this world. All sickness, all rebellion against God and violation of His expectations, all evil, all deception, all immorality, all violation of God's expectations, etc. In God's kingdom all these things are turned around through Jesus and will be eventually eliminated.

It's in this present conflict of kingdoms that we see values revealed—values of both kingdoms. The Kingdom

---

[51] "For he has rescued us from the kingdom of darkness and transferred us into the Kingdom of his dear Son..." (Colossians 1:13 NLT).

[52] "We know that we are children of God, and that the whole world is under the control of the evil one" (1 John 5:19).

[53] "Satan, who is the god of this world, has blinded the minds of those who don't believe. They are unable to see the glorious light of the Good News. They don't understand this message about the glory of Christ, who is the exact likeness of God" (2 Corinthians 4:4 NLT).

"You used to live in sin, just like the rest of the world, obeying the devil—the commander of the powers in the unseen world. He is the spirit at work in the hearts of those who refuse to obey God" (Ephesians 2:2 NLT).

of God has positive, loving, right, encouraging, and uplifting values.

However, each of these positive values is opposed by the kingdom of darkness. You and I experience the ramifications of this on a daily basis. (Sounds like *Lord of the Rings*, doesn't it?)

Actually, the kingdom of Satan has nothing positive to offer. All he and his kingdom can do is try to negate that which is positive in the Kingdom of God. "The thief [Satan] comes to steal, and to kill, and to destroy." Those are Jesus' words in John 10:10.

Therefore, regarding the value of health and healing, the Kingdom of God is totally "full health" for everyone. We could call this the "Kingdom of God universal health" plan. Here's a picture of that value as it exists in full measure in eternity, described in Revelation 21:3-4 (NLT):

> I heard a loud shout from the throne, saying, "Look, God's home is now among his people! He will live with them, and they will be his people. God himself will be with them. He will wipe every tear from their eyes, and there will be no more death or sorrow or crying or pain. All these things are gone forever."

Notice that in God's kingdom, where He is present, there is no suffering. All pain or crying caused by sickness, disease, suffering, and death are gone because those things no longer exist—and never did in God's kingdom. They exist only in the kingdom of this world.

Therefore, at this time in our world, the kingdom of darkness opposes God and brings sickness, pain, suffering, and ultimately death to the planet.

And unfortunately for us, the kingdom of the evil one now controls our planet. That's why bad things happen to good people. And why good things happen to bad people.

"We know that we are children of God, and that the whole world is under the control of the evil one" (1 John 5:19).

So when Jesus came the first time 2,000 years ago as a "Lamb," He started the revolution to once again implement His kingdom values on the earth and roll back the power of Satan. And that was definitely true about the kingdom value of health and healing.

When we read the four stories about Jesus in the New Testament (The Gospels of Matthew, Mark, Luke, and John), we quickly observe Jesus healed people who came to Him, day in and day out in various and many ways.

If we move into the fifth book of the New Testament, the book of the Acts of the Apostles, we see stories of those who followed Him who healed others in His name.

His name has power in it because He is the all-powerful Son of God, the King, who's resurrected! Since He is the Almighty, the Creator of Heaven and Earth,[54] and the One who loves those He made, why wouldn't healing be part of His nature?[55]

So I've discovered through my own battle with cancer, there's a strong connection between (1) health, (2) sickness,

---

[54] "For in him all things were created: things in heaven and on earth, visible and invisible, whether thrones or powers or rulers or authorities; all things have been created through him and for him" (Colossians 1:16).

[55] "This is how God's love was revealed among us: God sent His one and only Son into the world, so that we might live through Him. [10] And love consists in this: not that we loved God, but that He loved us and sent His Son as an atoning sacrifice for our sins" (1 John 4:9-10).

and (3) healing by the powerful hand of Jesus, who is also Jehovah Rapha of the Old Testament.

I've gained in my understanding of how these three things intersect for the follower of the Messiah as I've wrestled with how to rid my body of the esophageal cancer.

Jesus healed when He was on Earth, and I believe He's still implementing that value of health today in our world since He's the living Lord and loves all people.

How we experience His healing hand today is a question that deserves to be wrestled with. And as we wrestle, a number of other questions arise about this area of healing as well. Some questions may have answers and some may remain a mystery.

And we must realize many theologians and philosophers in the Christian church today have differing views on how this reality works, or if it's a reality at all. So studying this issue, or even considering Jesus' healing reality today, is not a "slam dunk" issue.

I can only share my experience and thoughts on how I view it and have wrestled with this subject, and hope they are helpful to others in a way that brings them closer to the God of healing, Jehovah Rapha.

More of my thinking on health and healing is found in Chapters 10 and 11, where I've reposted some blogs I wrote over the past three years while sitting in the cancer eclipse darkness. Hopefully from these some mental darkness is lifted for us and not a lot of new darkness is created!

10

HOW IS GOD INVOLVED WITH US WHEN WE'RE SICK?

This is a good question and one raised to me often during the past three years. When I was healthy the question never crossed my mind.

The length of my cancer fight, however, gave me pause to raise these questions and muse over issues that were outside the realm of my experience for seventy years.

Because God is outside of time and space, above and beyond us in every way and clothed in mystery, it is difficult to speak with any certainty and clarity to this issue of His involvement.

One certainty I did reach over these three years is the fact that God, as Jehovah Rapha, heals today in several ways—through the power created in our bodies, through allopathic medicine, through naturopathic medicine, and supernaturally, by a "divine touch."

And my belief is that Jesus, as the Creator and One who holds all things together, has His healing hand somehow involved in all of the healing ways applied to sickness. He's Jehovah Rapha. No doctor is.

Some doctors acknowledge that biblical fact while others do not. Recognition, however, does not change spiritual reality.

Which method He chooses is up to Him. And as we'll see, not everyone gets healed today for several reasons. This, of course, raises more questions, and often there are no satisfying answers.

Nevertheless, if we are healed or not, at a minimum God wants us to come to Him in the name of Jesus and ask to be healed from cancer or any other disease or sickness we have.

Jesus' name is unique and powerful, as we saw in the last chapter, and as Philippians 2:9-11 indicates

Therefore, God elevated Him to the place of highest honor and gave Him the Name above all other names, that at the Name of Jesus every knee should bow, in heaven and on earth and under the earth, and every tongue confess that Jesus Christ is Lord, to the glory of God the Father.

If we already believe in Him, He's waiting to work with us and walk with us in our health situation or any other situation of interest to us. Our interest becomes His interest because He's a loving father.

If we don't believe in Him, He loves us anyway and is waiting for us to come to Him for His love and healing. Maybe this health crisis you're facing will put you on the wonderful path of experiencing God's presence and touch in the midst of the pain.

And if you think you're not good enough to go to Jesus—don't worry—none of us are good enough! Jesus didn't come to help and rescue "good people." He came to help and rescue those of us who know we've got issues in our lives and need some outside help.

Friendships Count

One of the tremendous benefits to us in our cancer eclipse was the many friends we know who were praying for us. We are part of a group of thirty couples, all of whom believe in Jesus and believe in the power and reality of prayer to God the Father.

Each time I sent out a blog post they would pray for us. Looking back, their support in this way, as well as the personal encouragement to press forward, stabilized our journey.

Some people who go through suffering and crisis are very private. I chose to be open and transparent about my cancer battle. Sometimes I would think, "I've got to stop sharing what I'm going through and thinking about because conversations with friends are all about me much of the time."

However, in hindsight, there was a great personal advantage in that for me: it was the wonderful support and regular prayers to God for healing and the help we received from others. For me, this advantage totally outweighed the idea of suffering in silence and alone.

I can't quantify how much this contributed to my physical healing, but it certainly made a great difference in my mental health and perseverance. I would definitely recommend finding a strong, loving support group for anyone going through a cancer battle!

Meditations Throughout the Journey

Rather than reinvent the wheel on some of my thinking on this subject, I'm sharing here content from my blog, www.GrissenCancerJourney.com. These posts were sent out as I went through the cancer eclipse.

These articles represent summary thoughts of the spiritual and personal aspects of fighting cancer when I was in that direct battle from September 2014 through 2017. Yes, I'm still healing as I move into 2018.

Living with a Spiritual Reality—Not Everyone Gets Healed

I define "divine" or "supernatural" healing as a supernatural act by God, the Father, in the name of Jesus, the Messiah, through the power of the Holy Spirit, which immediately resolves a physical, emotional, or spiritual problem we are carrying.

Approximately one-fifth of the Gospel narrative is devoted to Jesus' healing ministry. At the start of His ministry, Jesus "went throughout Galilee, teaching in their synagogues, preaching the good news of the kingdom, and healing every disease and sickness among the people" (Matthew 4:23).

This was a supernatural working of Christ, with no doctors, hospitals, or equipment involved. Presently the Christian church has different views on whether Jesus is still supernaturally healing today or not. And we do periodically have some legitimate concern about "faith healers" and their credibility.

But one observation I've made over the years about divine or supernatural healing is, those who believe in it see

God heal in this way, and those who don't believe in it aren't experiencing or seeing God's healing touch in this way. Why is that? Could it be "Ask and you shall receive" (Matthew 7:7)?

Recently I've read a book called *God's Generals — The Healing Evangelists*, by Robert Liardon. These are biographies of five "faith healers" living during my lifetime. All of them were involved in the Pentecostal Christian movement, and according to written and verbal reports, they saw many people supernaturally healed through a "touch" of God's power.

Since my religious background was not within Pentecostalism, these biographies gave me a new appreciation for this part of the Christian church and new insights into God's divine healing ways.

One of those faith healers was Oral Roberts, a part-Native American Oklahoman, born to poor, committed Christian parents on January 24, 1918. Not without controversy surrounding him all of his ministry life, Roberts started out with a powerful preaching and healing tent ministry to tens of thousands in the 1950s.

He established the largest Christian university in the world in the 1960s. In the 1970s he started a television ministry that reached millions. And he and his wife, Evelyn, suffered much controversy and personal tragedy in the 1980s.

Here's an illustration, from the book, of one crusade where deaf children were healed.

The first place Oral used his Canvas Cathedral was in Durham, N.C., a city that welcomed him with open arms. Although the tent could seat three thousand, on many nights, there were as many as nine thousand people in attendance.

Oral could see overflow crowds that would encircle the outside of the tent to listen. He was overwhelmed by the response and kept his eyes on the Lord to give him the message for the people.

Each night while he was in Durham, a small number of deaf children from the local school for the deaf were brought to the meetings. And, each night, as Oral prayed for a different group of these children, their ears were opened to sounds and words; some could suddenly hear the music.

The crowd was electrified—and so was Oral! Many of those sweet, deaf children received a complete healing and were able to both hear and speak, moving the crowds to cry tears of joy. Those whose ears were not completely healed could hear sounds that were not possible for them to hear before.[56]

Yet even healing evangelist Oral Roberts did not see everyone healed! Here's how he lived with that:

In later years, Oral would admit there were things about God's healing power that he didn't understand. While he expected everyone whom he touched with his right hand to be healed, some were not. (At the beginning of his ministry, God told him to use his right hand to touch those who needed healing.)

---

[56] Robert Liardon, *God's Generals—The Healing Evangelists*, Whitaker House, 1030 Hunt Valley Circle, New Kensington, PA. 15068, 2011, page 184.

He simply learned to follow the Lord in obedience and pray in faith for everyone who came to him for prayer. He came to understand that the power was God's, the healing was Gods, and the ministry was God's.[57]

Why isn't everyone healed when they seek healing? Oral Roberts didn't know, and I'm not sure I ever heard a good reason for that either.

Here are several thoughts I've had on the subject as I continue reflecting on it. Send me your thoughts at CancerEclipse@gmail.com

One reason may be enshrouded in the mystery of God's will. While it would be encouraging for God to heal everyone who asks, it may also be merciful in some way known only to Him, that not everyone is healed. We don't know the eternal, hidden purposes and will of God. We can only submit to Him here and now, in time and space.

Another reason might be in the reality of the present spiritual battle being waged between the Kingdom of God and the kingdom of darkness. We gain insight into this battle in the book of Daniel when his prayers were not answered for three weeks because of the spiritual battle being waged.[58]

---

[57] Ibid., pg. 183.

[58] "Don't be afraid, Daniel. Since the first day you began to pray for understanding and to humble yourself before your God, your request has been heard in heaven. I have come in answer to your prayer.

"But for twenty-one days the spirit prince of the kingdom of Persia blocked my way. Then Michael, one of the archangels,

This means realities even in the supernatural realm are not static but fluid. Those of us in the material realm cannot see these dynamics in the spiritual realm since they're carried out beyond our senses. But this reality could have some implications for supernatural healing of which we are unaware, as Daniel was unaware why his prayer was not answered for twenty-one days.

A third reason could simply relate to the imperfection of our world. Full healing comes with the new body and the full entrance of God's kingdom at the end of time. Until then, the imperfections, power plays, and spiritual maneuverings going on could somehow affect full healing for everyone now.

Cancer Clarifies Our Mortality

Cancer clarifies and highlights the reality of our mortality and raises the issue of immortality. As I faced my upcoming demise, my thoughts naturally moved beyond that truth to what comes after the grave.

And the reality of mortality and promise of immortality impact my prayers for healing — a subject I'm wrestling with much these days on this cancer journey. Since something is going to take me to the grave, should I even pray for healing? Healing the body is a temporal reality anyway.

For example, Lazarus, with his miraculous resurrection, still ended up in the grave a second time, in need of the final resurrection. (His story is in the Gospel of John, chapter 11.)

---

came to help me, and I left him there with the spirit prince of the kingdom of Persia. Now I am here to explain what will happen to your people in the future, for this vision concerns a time yet to come" (Daniel 10:12-13 NLT).

If we are healed from some sickness, the best we can do is get a few more years on this planet without the disease that caused us to cry out for healing in the first place. And then a recurrence or a second disease might hit us and finish our life. At least for 100% of us, something will!

It almost makes me want to just "take the hits" as they come and agree with Solomon in Ecclesiastes 2:17, "… all of it is meaningless, a chasing after the wind."

Yet my natural desire is to gain more time here to spend with Sheri, family, and friends and to make some positive difference in the lives of a few people.

How would you use more days if you got them?

I'm sure Lazarus was thankful for more time with his family and friends as well.

So when it comes to prayers for healing, how does all this shake out?

Based on Lazarus' example, we might say that healing is a valid and powerful aspect of the <u>Kingdom of God</u>. We also realize his healing demonstrated the <u>compassion of Jesus</u> for Lazarus, his sisters, and friends. And in Lazarus' example, we discover the reason behind Lazarus' miracle: <u>the glory of God</u>.

Perhaps those are three major elements of any physical healing on this planet—God's compassion expressed through Kingdom healing for His glory.

When we hear the "C" word, or something else as ominous, perhaps the first thoughts we should take to God are: "Is this affliction unto death, or is it for some other purpose?" "What are you doing in my life now?"

Our subjective understanding of God's intention for our life on this point will move our prayers in one of two directions:

- If we sense it's unto death, then we want to pray for courage and perseverance in faith as we move toward the threshold of the next life.

  We also need to ensure our house is in order — and that's something wise to have in place anyway since we are all mortal and don't know the day of our demise.

- If it's not unto death, then I believe the courage to pray for healing is appropriate — as Peter said in the Gospel of John 6:68, "Lord, to whom shall we go? You have the words of eternal life." And beside eternal life, He also has the power to heal. Try to name one other person who does.

How am I seeing this for myself? When I first heard about my esophageal cancer and started praying about it, I didn't sense from God that cancer would take my life at this time. And now, as far as I can discern via PET scans, blood tests, and energy level, the cancer is gone, or at least in remission.

Through diet, exercise, supplements, etc., I'm doing everything in my power to keep it that way. Do I ever wonder if there's still a cancer cell in my body? Yes, I do.

But I'm not omniscient, and He is. Therefore, trust in His goodness and mercy is in order. And I'm thanking Him for healing and have more courage to pray that for others as well.

Is There a Connection Between Sin and Sickness?

In a prior post I mentioned the connection between sickness and death — is our sickness taking us to death, or not?

Yesterday in a personal meditation on the healing at the pool of Bethesda in The Gospel of John 5:1-15, I discovered a connection between sickness and sin. Is our sickness a result of our sin or not? What's your answer to that question?

Here's the Paraphrased Story …

The Pool of Bethesda was a "place of healing" in Jerusalem. Once each year, an angel stirred the waters, and the first one into the pool was healed. Competition ensued.

The lame man was one of many lame, blind, and paralyzed people gathered there waiting for that event to happen. However, he was not as fast as others and, therefore, faced defeat year after year.

His paralysis happened thirty-eight years before this time and from an unstated cause. Daily he was brought there by someone (must have had a sack lunch along) and was picked up again at night and taken home.

This was his daily routine and existence for those thirty-eight years. What a challenge for his caregivers!

I'm sure this pool party became quite a nice social outlet for the paralytics and other sick, and probably a support group at the same time. After thirty-eight years you must have some buddies laying there with you.

Fortunately for him, in his thirty-eighth year there, Jesus walked through the pool area and for some unstated reason focused on this man rather than any of the many others (at least to our knowledge).

Jesus talked with him about his background and then gave him three commands:
(1) Get up!
(2) Bend back down and pick up your mattress!
(3) Walk!

The man obeyed what Jesus asked and found his paralysis gone. He could get up. He could bend. He could lift and carry. He could walk away from the pool! Wow — and after thirty-eight years of paralysis! Finally victory! Finally healing!

All this happened with no strings attached, and the man didn't even know who the doctor was. Later he did connect again with Jesus, the Great Physician, but this time in the temple.

And there Jesus said an interesting thing to him: "See, you are well again." [Which means he was well before he was paralyzed.] "Stop sinning or something worse may happen to you." (v. 14)

My Thought...

Obviously, this man's paralysis happened because of some sin in his life. Sin is biblically defined as "missing God's target." We could also say sin is doing what we want that contradicts what God wants. Somehow in his youth, this man missed God's target, which then resulted in his paralysis either directly or indirectly.

Jesus, in His graciousness as a priest, dealt forgiveness to the man for his sin in the midst of the healing. Later in the temple Jesus gave him the warning: "Don't continue on in your sinful way or something worse than paralysis could happen to you!"

This would seem to show that when we are sick, we should discern if our sickness is a result of our erring ways that need to be straightened out or if there's some other cause. Perhaps a bad germ simply entered our body, making us sick, or we had an accident, or suffered from a natural catastrophe, or some combination.

In the Bible we see God uses sickness to get our attention and move our eyes and hearts back toward Him in faith and obedience. So reflection on the reason for our sickness is a valid and positive element of our faith walk and a wise exercise to do in our sick state.

I know with my cancer, that path has been one I've taken. I've considered my ways—my past, my present, and my future. Out of this reflection, there have been issues and actions in my life that I needed to talk with Jesus about. It's been a freeing path to walk. And it's been a strengthening path for my faith.

Not All Sickness is Unto Death, and Not All Sickness is the Result of Sin

Sin and sickness are also connected in James 5:14-15. "Is anyone of you sick? He should call the elders of the church to come and pray for him and anoint him with oil in the name of the Lord. And the prayer of faith will make the sick person well. And if they have sinned, they will be forgiven." Notice James says, "*if* they have sinned."

In John 9:2-3, Jesus clarifies that not all sickness is a result of sin: "And His disciples asked Him, 'Rabbi, who sinned, this man or his parents, that he would be born blind?' Jesus answered, 'It was neither that this man sinned, nor his parents; but it was so that the works of God might be displayed in him.'"

It seems there is JOY in any healing. But the WARNING from the paralytic's story and the passage in James is also there in any sickness: "See, you are well again. Stop sinning or something worse could happen to you!"

Should a King Go to Doctors?

One day during this cancer trek, as I tried to order my thoughts from a jumbled mass, I found this passage in 2 Chronicles 16:12, which summarizes a lesson I learned through my cancer eclipse: "In the thirty-ninth year of his reign, Asa developed a serious foot disease. Yet even with the severity of his disease, he did not seek the LORD's help but turned only to his physicians."

What's interesting to me about Asa is he had sought the Lord all of his life, yet at the end of it did not seek God in relationship to his foot disease.

Asa was one of the good kings of Judah, who reigned forty-one mostly peaceful years. Here are some positive statements in Asa's biography shared with us in 2 Chronicles 14:1-16:14.

Asa did what was good and right in the eyes of the Lord his God. (14:2)

He commanded Judah to seek the Lord, the God of their fathers, and to obey His laws and commands. (14:4)

Then Asa called to the Lord his God and said, "Lord, there is no one like you to help the powerless against the mighty" (14:11).

Azariah [a prophet] went out to meet Asa and said to him, "Listen to me, Asa, and all Judah and Benjamin. The Lord is with you when you are with him. If you seek him, he will be found by you, but if you forsake him, he will forsake you…" (15:2).

They entered into a covenant to seek the Lord, the God of their fathers, with all their heart and soul. (15:12)

They sought God eagerly, and he was found by them. So the Lord gave them rest on every side. (15:15)

Although he did not remove the high places from Israel, Asa's heart was fully committed to the Lord, all his life. (15:17)

For the eyes of the Lord range throughout the earth to strengthen those whose hearts are fully committed to him. (16:9)

Why did Asa—with all his positive background of seeking the Lord—not turn to God, Jehovah Rapha, the Healer, when he needed help with his foot disease? It was severe, and the implication from the passage is God would have helped him with it, but he didn't ask.

I can't answer that for Asa. But for myself I know I did the same thing with most of my ailments and those of loved ones throughout my seventy-three-plus years of life—I would turn to the doctors and the hospital treatments first, without even thinking about asking God for His hand of divine healing!

How could I be so arrogant, unthoughtful, and unthankful to God? Here's how:

- Human pride, bravado, self-reliance, and can-do spirit—the spirit of our nation. This creates the thought process: "I can visit doctors and the local hospital. Let's get over there and get it done!!!"

- We've got such a good medical establishment in the USA. My first thought is to go to the doctors for a diagnosis, medicine, or operation.

- I passively considered it was God doing the healing through the medical establishment anyway—which is a truth. After all, the doctors wouldn't be there if He hadn't created the laws of physics to use, the human brains to figure it out with our medical centers and procedures.

- That's how I was taught and trained by my parents— have a physical problem? Go visit Doc Smith to get it fixed. My first operation was a tonsillectomy at age eight, and Doc did it!

- In my religious background and training, we didn't put an emphasis on seeking the Lord for His divine hand of healing. We prayed for the sick generally, but the underlying assumption was God would do that through the doctors and not in some other, non-medical way.

Through my recent cancer journey, I saw this tendency and now act differently. Instead, I try to implement a knee-jerk reaction to seek Jehovah Rapha first when I have a physical need.

What's my report card on applying this thinking at this point? Probably a C+. Old habits die slowly!

Healing Raises Profound Questions About End-of-Life Issues

The blog post on King Asa garnered some very good feedback. One friend, Gordon, sent me a number of questions this topic raised for him. I would like to pass these on to you. They are very deep and good ones to contemplate, especially for those of us in our golden years.

Another book, written by a wiser person than I, is needed to answer them or at least wrestle competently with them. But please put on your thinking cap and let me know if you have any thoughts to these questions.

Dave, Thanks for sending us your thoughts on divine healing. They are very thought provoking. I appreciate the tie-in with Bible passages. This discussion raises some questions I'm thinking about in end-of-life issues. Here are a few of them …

- How should we think of assisted suicide? We go to the doctors all of our lives for healing of human ailments, take their advice and their medicines. If at the end of our lives we bear much pain, loss of bodily functions, etc., and God does not heal, and doctors can do no more, is it okay to go to the doctor and be assisted into eternal healing?

- When do we know when God is calling us home? Medical science can extend our lives today even though we've got no quality of life or hope of a cure. If I take advantage of these means to extend my life, is God calling me home but I'm using methods to refuse that in his timing?

- At age forty-nine, I ruptured a couple disks in my back and was in extreme pain for a year before getting worked into a rotation for back surgery. I did seek divine healing but didn't get it.

- Was God saying "no" to my healing, or was I suffering the consequences of being unsuccessful as a Christian and not deserving of his intervention? Or was He again calling me home but the docs prevented that?

- I have known people who have gone to faith healers seeking God's healing but not getting results. How does one get God to respond? When I started having hereditary heart problems with irregular heartbeats, I needed cardiac conversion on four occasions to keep me from having a probable heart attack. Another call by God to enter eternity that I refused?

- All through the years I was trying to follow God and be obedient, but He did not step in with supernatural or divine healing. Why?

- I also think of the branch of Christianity that only accepts divine healing and refuses medical treatment. They periodically end up in court in a lawsuit for letting a child die for lack of a common antibiotic because they believe God will intervene. Maybe sometimes God does intervene for them and we don't hear about it? We hear about the child who dies and the parents being hauled into court. This whole topic absolutely mystifies me.

- And of course, in the above scenario we have the interesting issue of the government's control over and in our lives. Should the government tell a parent they must send their child to a doctor? At what age does that stop? And who's the government anyway? It seems this would be a judge who might have a different bias on healing or faith or God and forces the parent against their conscience to do what they feel is right and best.

- On the other hand, I think I continually receive healing in the way God has designed my body to heal wounds, heal broken bones, heal colds and flus, etc. He does that for believers and non-believers alike. He does that for plants and animals, too.

- Healing appears to be built into our genetic code by Him. Is divine healing reserved for certain believers only, or are you aware of atheists or agnostics receiving divine healing? I've never even thought about that until now.

- I do not understand why God helps some and not others. When one experiences God's healing and utilizes prayer, nutritional interventions, medical treatments, which are all the treatments available, how is one certain which one is really working? At times it seems like there is some formula that one needs to get just right, but it proves illusive.

- It appears God uses many interventions: diet, medical science, physical exercise, obedience, and miracles in life, and we have to pay attention to them all and not neglect any. End-of-life issues are part of my fears. I dread end-of-life scenarios.

As you can see, this whole topic leaves me confused and frustrated because I cannot figure out why peoples' experiences vary so significantly regarding healing issues.

The Pain and Suffering of Sickness

Writing blogs about my cancer eclipse and thinking during that time has put me in touch with a lot of people who are also suffering from cancer and other diseases. Often I leave a conversation thinking, "They surely have it much worse than I do!"

Suffering in life is a reality. But a key issue in suffering is, how do we live with it, think about it, and deal with it?

Sickness and disease is one form of human suffering in our world. Not only do they cause physical pain, but also emotional pain as we wrestle with our condition in relationship to our weakening bodies being wracked by something negative.

Practically, we can suffer from a variety of causes. Here are some of those conditions which cause suffering:

1) experiencing results of *the fallen world*—disease, natural disasters, accidents,
2) experiencing negative results of *other's choices*,
3) experiencing pressures and even *martyrdom because we choose to do what's right*,
4) experiencing the consequences of our own *bad decisions*.

This suffering can be physical, emotional, psychological, and spiritual. In other words, suffering affects us holistically. My physical cancer hit me in certain ways in each of these areas. Yours probably does, too.

On the spiritual level, suffering can cause us spiritual lift or depressive pain, depending on how we live with an important, theological question: If God is sovereign, omnipotent, omniscient, good, and loving—why does he let me suffer and not stop it? Why did He allow this negative to hit my life in the first place?

As my late friend Walt Henrichsen once said in regard to Job, "Why does God sometimes treat His friends like His enemies? We simply don't know." And Steve Estes said this on the issue, "God permits what He hates to accomplish what He loves."

But this reality does cause us some spiritual pain, and hopefully some spiritual growth as well. Only faith in His character (all of those characteristics mentioned above) allows us to live with these pains and move forward with trust and joy and a deeper relationship with God.

11
ENCOURAGEMENT IN THE MIDST OF THE CANCER ECLIPSE

How to Deal with a Negative Medical Report

On September 30, 2014, through a CT scan, I discovered I had esophageal cancer. This was definitely a heavy negative medical report for me!

Then on October 17, 2014, Sheri discovered her cancer was back. This was another negative medical report.

The only positive in this picture was we were battling this crazy stuff together. We could both sit in our easy chairs with our feet up, feel bad at the same time, and fight over who gets the coffee—at least Keurig would make it.

As these types of negative medical reports were hitting us regularly, I read Psalm 112:7 in the Bible. "The one who trusts in God need not fear a bad report, for his heart is UNSHAKEN, since he trusts in the LORD." (ISV, emphasis mine)

If we personalize this, we could say, "The cancer patient who trusts in God...will have an UNSHAKEN inner core."

Sheri and I often felt shaken on our cancer journeys. There's much in them to shake us up to the core, isn't there?

But for us God provided the counterpoint to all of these personal tremors. Since He's the only stable point in life when things go bad, trust in Him to get us through the shaking is the solution. Trust creates stability at our core.

We are then "unshaken" by our bad reports.

And one final Psalm reference on this topic from Psalm 112:7-8, "[The cancer patient] will have no fear of bad news; his heart is steadfast, trusting in the Lord. His heart is secure; he will have no fear. In the end he will look in triumph on his foes."

Re-Thinking Cancer? About Time?

As we walked our cancer journey in 2015, we discovered the historical conflict existing today between allopathic and naturopathic medicine, which is still an active one. [Note: I wrote more extensively on this issue in Chapter 5.]

The history is very negative, but there may be hope on the horizon the two could be integrated to actually give cancer patients more help than in the past. (And we'll know that happened when our health insurance covers naturopathic treatments as well as allopathic treatments.)

In his weekly blog www.Bio-Flourish.com, Dr. Mark Wagner, a medical doctor studying naturopathy and nutrition, reviewed a new book about re-thinking cancer and treatment: *Tripping Over the Truth* by Travis Christofferson.

Here's his post and review on *The Return of the Metabolic Theory of Cancer Illuminates a New and Hopeful Path to a Cure*. Mark writes:

> I spent last week in Mexico with my father-in-law. He's a cancer survivor. I can't tell you how wonderful

it was to see grandpa looking so well, interacting with his grandchildren, and enjoying the tropical sun. This time last year he had no hair, no energy, and he shivered a lot.

Fortunately, his cancer is one of the few types that responds well to the standard slash and burn approach to cancer therapy: chemo and radiation. I realize other people are not so lucky.

So it was fitting this week that I should read *Tripping Over the Truth* by Travis Christofferson. The book is a *tour de force* exposé on what is both so right and so wrong with cancer research today—or any research for that matter, where big money and consensus reality drives the conversation long past its expiration date.

We are in the midst of a massive re-think on cancer. A brilliant cluster of researchers is starting to see cancer not so much as a genetic disease, but as a metabolic disease. Which means it may be easier and cheaper to treat than we were able to imagine while under the spell of complex genomes and fabled genetic cures.

Even the venerable James Watson himself (he of double-helix fame) has recently changed his tune, admitting that the Somatic Mutation Theory of cancer (and the mega $billions spent on it) has yielded surprisingly little in the way of useful therapeutic information and that it is time to look elsewhere. Watson says, "We must focus much, much more on the wide range of metabolic and oxidative vulnerabilities of cancer."

In other words, it's time to focus on what we are feeding cancer. On what kinds of food and molecules might disrupt the unique and relatively simple metabolism of cancer, regardless of its bewildering, catch-me-if-you-can, unpredictable and manifold genomes.

This book, a five-star read, is almost like a detective novel in places. In fact, it is so accessible and well written, that I often found myself thinking I should just give up trying to do science writing myself, because maestros like Christofferson have got it covered.

So do yourself a favor and take a day or two off over the holidays to enjoy this book. Catch a glimpse of what could be a much better future for you, for your loved ones, and for all of us.

You can order this book here and support the non-profit Life Impact, Inc., at the same time. This is the organization Sheri and I started to provide care for international Christian workers. Just type the URL below in your browser, and the book will show up!

https://smile.amazon.com/Tripping-over-Truth-Overturning-Entrenched/dp/1603587292/ref=sr_1_1?s=books&ie=UTF8&qid=1505856917&sr=1-1&keywords=christofferson.

Is This a "Sign" Communicating Anything?

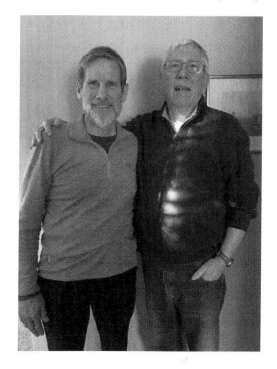

Does the light in this picture look coincidental? Do you want my opinion?

I'm standing by a wall in our living room with Tom Landis, a friend who had esophageal surgery two years before me for the same cancer. He's been a help and encouragement to me with his survival post-surgery advice, as well as providing answers to my questions about it.

On this visit to our home, pre-operation for me, I wanted to have a picture taken with him. Amazingly, light was shining through our blinds at that specific moment to hit my throat and abdomen in the exact locations where the esophagectomy would take place on March 14, 2017. (I've got scars in those locations now, post-op!)

Was this a coincidence or something more—like a "God-happening" to encourage me?

I tend to think it was an encouraging sign from Jesus, the Healer, that I'm in good hands for whatever came up in my operation. What do you think?

I look at it this way because the astronomical chances of all the following details falling randomly into place are higher than the national lottery! Maybe one of you mathematicians can figure out the odds with a powerful computer?

Here are the factors …

- The sun had to be shining that afternoon. (Not too difficult in Bend since we get 300 days of sunshine a year. But that afternoon could also have been one of the cloudy sixty-five!)

- The sun had to be in that exact location at that exact time. Ten minutes later and no shine!

- The blinds had to be set at the right angle to let the sun shine in. I did that randomly at 8:00 a.m.

- The blinds had to be at the right angle to let the light shine exactly on those spots instead of either too high or too low on my chest.

- The sun had to be at the right location to shine brightly on these spots rather than more to the right or the left on my chest.

- I had to be standing on Tom's left instead of vice versa, and in the right spot. I wasn't posing. This stance was random. (And if I was a couple inches shorter, it would have hit my mouth!)

- Tom and Madeleine, his wife, had to decide to leave at this exact time in their visit and then to discuss taking a picture.

- We had to make the decision to take the picture, get out the camera, decide on the location, move to that spot and line up — at the exact few minutes of time when the sun would be shining at that exact spot.

- Isn't it almost supernaturally bright for 2:30 p.m. on a winter afternoon?

- And finally — the BIG picture. The universe itself had to be lined up in exactly the right place in all of its facets and phases in order for this to create all of the above at this time. A different day in a different season, and the light would have hit at a different spot, if at all! Wow!

I'm not sure if and what God was communicating through this. Was it that I'm supernaturally healed through His power and light? (My final opportunity to check out this possibility was March 9 with the pre-op PET scan.)

Or perhaps that I would be totally okay going through the surgery on Tuesday, March 14?

At the very least, this was a tremendous encouragement to me at the time, and I still look at the picture today (post-op) with thankfulness for my path of healing. This picture went with me into my recovery room as well, with a "showing" to Dr. Oelschlager and some of his staff.

1 John 1:5 says, "This is the message we have heard from him and declare to you: God is light; in him there is no darkness at all."

James 1:17 says, "Every good and perfect gift is from above, coming down from the Father of the heavenly lights, who does not change like shifting shadows."

Psalm 97:11 says, "Light is risen to the just, and joy to the right of heart." (Douay-Rheims version)

Feeling Like I'm on Death Row!

One last day before the surgery

I feel like a man on death row, choosing my last meal this noon (a steak dinner?) and then waiting until I can be hooked up on the table tomorrow, go under, hopefully to rise again from the table later that day! (That's the $64,000 question based on a 9% national, 30-day operation survival rate average.)

This morning in my Bible reading, Psalm 91 was on the docket. Just what I needed! What a tremendous psalm of encouragement for someone facing the major esophagectomy—or any challenge for that matter. Here are my thoughts on God's thoughts revealed in this song.

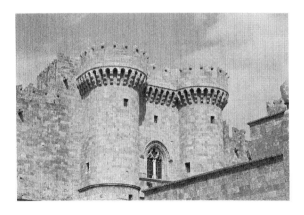

"He who dwells in the shelter of the Most High will rest in the shadow of the Almighty." (v. 1) This is a good place to be

when you hoist yourself up on the operating table. I think my soul will be "resting" tomorrow in that process. (I hate the air mask, however. That's where claustrophobia hits!)

"I will say of the Lord, 'He is my refuge and my fortress, my God, in whom I trust.'" (v. 2) This is my confession also—today, tomorrow, and the next day, on into eternity.

"Surely He will save you from...the deadly pestilence." (v. 3) Cancer is definitely deadly, and it surely is a pest—one created by our own bodies, unfortunately, but a pest, none-the-less. It will be nice to be saved from it either here or there.

"He will cover you with his feathers, and under his wings you will find refuge; his faithfulness will be your shield and rampart." (v. 4) Protection is needed in an operation, and protection is promised.

"You will not fear...the terror of the night...nor the pestilence that stalks in the darkness ..." (v. 5-6) Because of my preoccupation with the terribleness of the operation and the disabilities I might have afterwards, some fear has crept into my thoughts. (And the nights in the hospital were bad.)

Two days ago, I decided to focus on the "outcomes" rather than the "inputs." Here's my focus now: When I wake up on Tuesday afternoon after the operation, my cancer will be external to my body! That's a great outcome for extending my life—all the cancer we could see is gone!

"'Because he loves me,' says the Lord, 'I will rescue him; I will protect him, for he acknowledges my name.'" (v. 14) I do love the Lord to some degree. It's not easy to judge how much love is there since love can be expressed selfishly in a relationship, i.e., I love because of what I receive.

But I certainly acknowledge His name and will continue to do that no matter the outcome. I'm looking forward to the promise of protection and being rescued from this pestilence!

"He will call upon Me, and I will answer him. I will be with him in trouble. I will deliver him ..." (v. 15) We have been calling on Him for supernatural healing so an operation would not be necessary. His answer was, "Take the operation." So now I need to call on Him for deliverance in and through the operation.

"Trouble" and the need for "deliverance" indicates life is not a bed of roses or a box of chocolates, as Forest Gump indicated. So in the midst of this cancer trouble in which I find myself, I expect to wake up tomorrow afternoon and be delivered from this pestilence through the operation.

"With long life will I satisfy him and show him my salvation." (v. 16) How does one understand this? Many who follow God die at a young age. The Bible indicates seventy years is a solid lifespan, or eighty if one is strong. (Psalm 90:10)

I've already had seventy-three wonderful years of life. My bucket list is complete except for a visit to Israel. Staying around longer for the enjoyment of family and friends, and to have a positive impact on them with my life, is a wonderful wish and worthy goal, I think.

But what does God mean by, "I'll satisfy him with a long life?" I understand this to mean enjoy each day we have and be a positive presence in that particular day and hope I make it to eighty!

[Note Post-Operation: I experienced the truths of this Bible song [psalm] in many ways after my operation, as I note in the next post regarding a Red Sea experience.]

Delivered from Another "Red Sea" Experience

In reflection on my six-day operation, I realize how God took me through another Red Sea experience – a difficult time which came out positive. (The first time was the radiation-chemo treatments in 2014.)

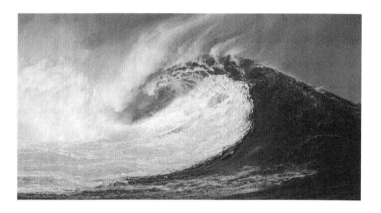

What Did I Experience?

- An **excellent epidural** without any side-effects or serious implications. A nurse said, "You have one of the best epidurals I've seen. They don't all look as good as yours."

- That epidural controlled my chest pain throughout my time without problems or spinal fluid leakage. In fact, I experienced **no post-op pain**.

- After pain meds were stopped, I experienced **no pain** after that to this day.

- Dr. Oelschlager, his team of doctors, and the nurses were amazed at my daily progress, so I was **released a day early**.

- I was encouraged as I heard one of the **assisting doctors was praying** for me during the operation.

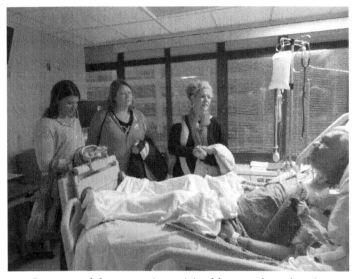

Just out of the operation, visited by my three lovely daughters!

- **Sheri was a shining presence** in my room each day, bringing me out of the stupor of the medications. Our **three daughters** all came to cheer me on—how I love them all!

- The **critical barium test** to check for throat leakage came back positive. My new esophagus would hold!

God has taken me through another Red Sea experience and I'm thankful to Him, as the Israelites were after their deliverance from an overwhelming situation:

> The Lord is my strength and my song; he has become my salvation. He is my God, and I will praise him, my father's God, and I will exalt Him…Your right

hand, O Lord, was majestic in power. Your right hand, O Lord, shattered the enemy (Exodus 15:2, 6).

Some Lessons from the Journey!

❖ The prayers of God's people make a difference.

Exactly how prayer works is a mystery to me, but then, God Himself is a mystery! We sensed the power of prayer in our lives as friends prayed.

❖ Medical technology & treatment are God's gifts.

These medical gifts make a difference in our lives in so many other ways, as well as in cancer situations.

❖ Our bodies have tremendous healing power.

God created huge power for healing within our bodies. If we allow our bodies to function well, we experience a wonderful plus factor in our health. This is the issue I've been harping on of food, toxins, health, and exercise, all of which affect our immune system.

In my case, the chemo-radiation taken at the end of 2014 dampened my cancer and caused it to mutate slightly. Then I went on a natural treatment path, instead of surgery, for two years.

Looking back, we see the natural path controlled and contained the cancer in a positive way although not eradicating it. The cancer was either too powerful, or I didn't take enough time on the natural track to see the tumor shrink and disappear.

In retrospect, this shows me the power of what we eat and how we treat our bodies. I suggest those who want to prevent cancer and those who are fighting cancer give serious attention to the food factors below.

The underlying principle in these factors is the elimination of toxins.

1) *Eliminate* as much sugar and sodium from our diet as we can—not an easy task.
2) *Eat organic* chicken and sausage.
3) *Eat organic* at least for the "dirty dozen." This eliminates fertilizer and weed killing toxins from our bodies. Why ask your immune system to fight those when it needs to fight cancer-forming cells and other diseases?
   Get the "dirty dozen" list from this URL:
   (http://www.myelomacrowd.org/fruits-veggies-buy-organic-dirty-dozen-clean-ten/?gclid=CLPW6K2_l9MCFZFafgodY7sDXQ)
4) *Drink smoothies or juices.* We drink a kale-blueberry-orange juice smoothie four or five times a week. We also drink a carrot-apple-onion-garlic-broccoli-radish-ginger root-beet juice four times a week.
   These strengthen the immune system and reportedly target cancer cells.
5) *Eat grass fed beef* and not too often. (The colon is aggravated by red meat. On our changed diet, my latest colonoscopy indicated a tract free of pre-cancerous polyps. I always had some removed before with each procedure.)
6) *Eat fresh caught, wild fish* not the farmed ones. As our waters continue to be more and more polluted, there's much more about fish and toxicity one can learn and apply.

Chris Wark. If you're fighting cancer and want another example of natural food impact to heal it, check out Chris Wark. His story is credible.

He was twenty-two years old when he got cancer. After an operation to remove a tumor from his colon, he chose not to have radiation and chemo, but learn how to build up his immune system and fight off further cancer in that way. (www.chrisbeatcancer.com)

He was able to do that through a very tough regimen of natural processes. This approach is not easy and takes much discipline. But Chris' wisdom is valuable for us today in the toxic environment in which we live and operate 24/7.

As you can see, our personal cancer journey has produced a philosophy of BOTH-AND. We need the established medical wisdom and treatments as well as the natural wisdom and treatments. Those two elements are a powerful double-barreled shotgun, leveled at any cancer we might develop.

The hand of God in our lives works through all of the above according to His will for each of us individually.

Thanks To "Operation Pioneers!"

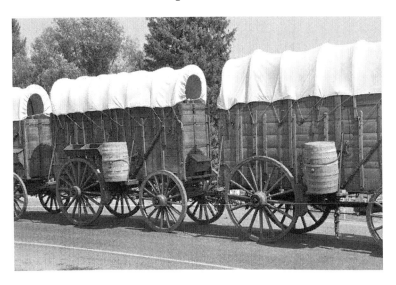

The other night I woke with the thought: "What if I had been the first one to have this operation? What if I was an "Operation Pioneer?"

Then when the cancer was discovered, some sharp surgeon (Ivor Lewis, to be exact) would say to me, "Dave, I think we can get the cancer out IF we take out your esophagus. Would you like to give that a try?"

If I was moving steadily and quickly toward the cemetery anyway, I would probably say "Yes, I'll be the guinea pig or rat, but what are the implications?"

The doc would say, "The risks you face are these:"

- We might cut something in there that would be hard to repair since I've never done this before.

- You might lose your voice, we're not sure how that would go. But you could learn sign language in that case.

- We hope we can resection your stomach to function as your new esophagus.

- We don't know if there will be leakage when we connect your stomach to the remainder of your esophagus tube. In fact, we're not quite sure how to do that exactly, but I'll give it a heroic try! I'd probably try tough, slim string since we haven't invented a good staple gun yet.

- We can't guarantee you will be able to eat. We think so, but we're not sure. You may have to be on a feeding tube for the rest of your life—and we hope that will be many years.

- And if you do survive the operation and recovery and are able to eat, we're not sure what food you'll tolerate or how much at a time. You may have to survive on Jell-o or yogurt.

- Oh, and by the way, you might not wake up. We don't have any statistical track record of success or failure since you are establishing it. So after your operation, our post-op survival rate will either be 100% survive or 100% don't.

- If all else fails, we can always throw a "Hail Mary!" We'll try everything we can think of in your operation and hope something works.

Fortunately, I was not the first one to have the operation, or the second or the third. Actually, in my case, they've been doing esophagectomies for years, improving procedures year by year.

So my expectations were very high that I'd come through in good shape, be able to eat, heal, and live a somewhat normal life afterwards. And fortunately, I'm on that track!

But I want to take my hat off and salute all those who were the first ones to be operated on for ALL types of operations!

They are truly Operation Pioneers and should be thanked by all of us for their courage and commitment to be at the head of the operation line. They basically did it for us, and we are thankful!

12
FINAL REFLECTIONS ON MY CANCER ECLIPSE

As I come to the three-year point from the time my cancer was first discovered and have taken the path I've described in this book, friends have raised good questions I've pondered.

In this chapter I want to try and clearly answer those questions with my current reflections. I want to stay on a growing curve, however, so some of these will undoubtedly change and develop as time goes on.

In Hindsight, Would I Do the Operation Again?

Since the operation itself went well for me, I wouldn't hesitate to do it again. If it hadn't gone well, I'm not sure what I would say since the operation is a "quality of life" as well as a survival issue.

Once we put our "hand to the plow" and decide to have the operation, we can't go back. So we do and will live with whatever consequences come for us from this direction.

In my case, I feel all things went exceptionally well. I'm eternally grateful for that. Someone else, however, for whatever reasons, may have a more difficult time. Hindsight is 20/20.

If someone gets esophageal cancer, it will be a decision that must be made pro or con if the cancer has not metastasized. If the cancer has spread, the operation is off the table as an option. (Then you should consider other options—heroic naturopathic or a treatment like John Jankuski did; see Appendix A.)

If the cancer does re-emerge for me, I'll probably second guess myself initially:

- Did the cancer get kicked into gear through oxygen introduced through the operation?

- Were some cells dropped in the operation that started growing?

- Did the operation or previous treatments weaken my immune system to such an extent my body couldn't overcome the cells that were left?

- Could I have overcome the cancer without an operation if I had hit it harder with natural treatments from the beginning? One friend beat a Stage IV cancer for seven years with prayer and the natural. (See Roy Bennet's story in Appendix A.)

At the same time, because of the way I processed my treatments every step of the way, I have a clear conscience I did the best I could with the information and thinking I had. I think that's the best we can do, looking forward.

Along the way I was open to counsel and advice although I knew I had to make my own decision about the path forward. It was no one else's decision to make, and I would be the one living with the consequences of whatever path I chose anyway, including this one.

So I wanted to choose well. I did not want to leave the decision to someone else and play the victim later.

But one "faith conviction" I have personally: I surely wouldn't want to have the operation without asking God for His guidance of the doctors all through the operation process and His healing hand on my life afterwards. I picture an operation as the doctor's hands being held by Jesus' hands as an operation progresses.

And I wouldn't want to have the operation without following His directive in the New Testament book of James:

> Is anyone among you sick? Let him call for the elders of the church, and let them pray over him, anointing him with oil in the name of the Lord. And the prayer of faith will save the one who is sick, and the Lord will raise him up. And if he has committed sins, he will be forgiven. Therefore, confess your sins to one another and pray for one another, that you may be healed. The prayer of a righteous person has great power as it is working (James 5:14-16 ESV).

It's very difficult for me to say any other factors contributed more to my operation's success than God's supervision of it, which is a faith statement, I realize.

Why Me? Why Did I Get Cancer?

"Cancer requires that I stumble around in the debris of dreams I thought I was entitled to and plans I didn't realize I had made." —Kate Bowler, cancer survivor[59]

The first question I asked myself when I found out the Stage II tumor existed in my esophagus was, "Why ME and why now?" I was just about retired and looking forward to a few good years of fun and travel with my wife. Now this? What a downer! What a discouragement! What a black hole! What a total eclipse of life by a dark reality!

As I step back from feeling like the victim with the "why me" and "why now" questions and start processing the practical reasons why cancer hit me, I realize the questions should be, "why not me?" and "why not now?"

At the time I was diagnosed with cancer I was seventy years old and had lived a long, healthy, and fulfilling life up to that point.

I worked for myself. I have a great family. I had some retirement money saved to add to my social security to live on. My bucket list was almost filled. (I would still love to visit Israel and experience an opera in New York at the Met, however.)

What else did I have to experience? I was at a point in life where every day was a dish of ice cream, a box of chocolates, or a bowl of cherries.

Who did I think I was that cancer should not affect me when more than one out of three people in the USA will fight cancer during their lifetime? I had a 38.5% chance of

---

[59] Kate Bowler is a Duke professor and cancer survivor. Her blog is (http://katebowler.com/blog/).

getting some type of cancer, and now with my diagnosis, I knew which group I was in. (That percentage is already 50% in the UK for some reason.)

So armed with this new perspective, 'cancer did happen to me for some reason,' I identified some <u>probable causes or factors</u> in my life which led to this reality.

The <u>first factor</u> I identified was a compromised immune system.

The physical fact is the body's immune system is naturally weaker and weaker over time as we age. Add to that reality the fact that toxins in our environment, absorbed in one way or another into our bodies, weaken us even further and more quickly.

In my case, I grew up on a farm where fertilizer residue blew out of bags into my nose on a continual basis. We would "dust" the fields with a poison to kill bugs, and although a mask was worn, it was impossible not to breathe some of that over time.

And then there was DDT. In the summer the enemy was large black flies filling up our garage in huge numbers. They needed elimination before they could move into our house. DDT was the agent to do the killing. And I was the human instrument to carry out the deed.

So the liquid would go into a hand pump container. Then all the doors and windows of the garage would be shut tight. I would start in one end of the garage pumping out the DDT into the air and moving around until the mist covered the whole room. This was all done WITHOUT wearing a mask. (Aren't we wiser today and much better stewards of our environment?)

In my childhood days and even into my forties and late fifties we had no idea how dangerous these chemicals were to the body. Did this type of childhood weaken my immune system so aberrant cells could grow later in life?

One caveat to this point: My father is now 100 years old, going on 101. He did all the stuff I did as well since I worked for him on the farm. How did his immune system get so much stronger? I had cancer when I was seventy. He's still going strong at 100 with no cancer!

The <u>second factor</u> that most likely affected my health situation and weakened my body is our American food chain.

Unfortunately, in the USA we have put dangerous toxins into our food chain through the fertilizers, weed killers, growth hormones, and bug killers we use to produce our crops and grow our animals.

This is done to ensure a bountiful crop, to create a more perfect looking fruit or vegetable, to increase the shelf life of produce in the supermarket, and to overall increase the financial bottom line for the farming industry.

After all, a farmer is in business to make money like anyone else. I was a young farmer once, raising celery in the 1950s and 60s; so I know.

There is not much we can do personally to counter this toxic direction today except to be aware of what foods we buy and eat and what issues are on the ballot.

When we're young, the immune system processes all these negative toxin inputs more easily. But over time, this also has a wearing effect on our body system. By the time I hit seventy, I'm sure my immune system was quite compromised.

More people today, especially the younger generation, purchase their fresh produce and some foodstuffs at stores selling organic and natural products.

This is a growing customer base in the USA, as Amazon recognized. Recently they invested 13.7 billion dollars to purchase Whole Foods and tap into this trend.

Another counter-cultural trend regarding food is the increase in personal gardening, even in cities where people are not landowners. More wooden boxes filled with rich earth serving as "fields" are being placed on balconies of apartment buildings or on their roofs.

(Piece of advice: If you're young and reading this, please consider changing your eating habits to eliminate as many toxins as possible. Do everything you can to keep your immune system strong!)

A third factor I identified was the diet I ate and my lack of understanding of the power of acid reflux.

Esophageal cancer often develops from a pre-cancerous state called Barrett's Syndrome. Barretts is caused by acid reflux. And acid reflux is caused by our diet.

In my case, the diet was heavy in fatty red meats, spicy foods, tomato paste and pizza, a daily glass of red wine later in life, and many carbs and sweets.

All of this added to my weight and created an acidic body and stomach. At one point in my mid-fifties, I was an unhealthy 230 pounds. Today my frame carries 165 pounds, and I'm feeling great.

Add to this the fact that my job often meant sitting in an office or driving around in a car, and without much exercise, I wasn't processing the fats or acid well.

And to top off the acid reflux issue, I discovered 80% of those who have it don't realize it. That was also my situation. I would sometimes experience a "TUMS night" when I ate pizza or other foods with tomato sauce. Otherwise, I was oblivious to the silent cancer producer.

My analysis of cancer-producing, immune-depleting factors identified a <u>fourth one</u>: our life lived in other countries.

During the 1970s and 80s we traveled much behind the Iron Curtain. In the 90s we traveled and lived in Central Asia. In both areas the food supply was either heavily fertilized or depleted of nutrition from years of use without fertilizers. Also, factories spewed out unfiltered smoke, lowering the air quality we breathed on a daily basis.

The <u>final</u> nail in the coffin was most likely stress. In cross-cultural moves, adjustments, and living, there is much stress our minds never recognize.

We moved to Vienna, Austria, in 1994 to train Christian leaders behind the Iron Curtain. Language school was a huge stress on me. Helping kids adjust to a different language, culture, and educational system was a stress. Traveling back and forth across communist borders was a stress. Once inside, operating 24/7 under watchful, KGB-type eyes was a stress.

Sheri and I came back to the USA after four years of that for our first home leave. I thought I was doing great and had adjusted just fine without much stress.

What I discovered was I didn't want to see people, make any new contacts, update our donors, or visit any groups or churches. I wanted to veg out. I was in a minor depression from stress.

In addition to the cross-cultural stress was also the stress created by our work generally. My career was mostly entrepreneurial and middle management. I had the privilege to start national and international projects and lead people in pursuit of objectives. There is some internal pressure in all of this even though the people I worked with were class acts and created very little stress!

When I put this whole picture together, I have quite a natural, physical, and medical rationale for answering the questions "Why Me and Why Now?"

Was I not a ticking cancer-candidate time bomb waiting to happen? Was not the cancer eclipse only a few weeks out on my calendar when I hit the age of seventy?

How Did I Apply James 5:14-18 and Seek Healing?

When my cancer eclipse happened and I heard the bad news I had esophageal cancer and then learned how devastating it is, the statistics were definitely scary. So I knew I was in some serious life trouble. My life had radically changed. My hopes about the future had been dashed. What should be my next steps?

Of course, listening to and tracking with my oncologist was the only option I knew at the time. Because we have such a wonderful medical establishment in this country, my default was to contact a doctor and do what they said.

When my cancer surfaced this was no exception. And the doctors along the way were all sincere and caring professionals, motivated to help me. What a privilege to have our medical establishment behind us.

Another Option to Fight Cancer...Prayer!

Normally when I had a headache, got the flu, or fought off a sore throat, I never considered going to God to ask Him for healing. But when cancer hit BIG TIME, I knew I needed some BIG TIME help outside of the ordinary if I was going to fight this and survive.

At that time, I remembered the Bible exhortation in James 5:14-16: "Is anyone among you sick? Let him call for the elders of the church, and let them pray over him, anointing him with oil in the name of the Lord. And the prayer of faith will save the one who is sick, and the Lord will raise him up."

My approach to the Bible has always been to read it as I would any book and let the context determine when something is not meant to be taken as literal.

For example, the text normally tips us off to poems, allegories, parables, visions, symbols, and other parts of speech that must be understand differently than as strictly written.

So the James passage seems to me to be a straight, literal exhortation to go to the elders of your local church to be prayed for when sick and hopefully raised up from the sickness.

In my circumstances, I surely wanted to be raised up from the cancer, and I knew Jesus has the power to do it. So based on this instruction, I put myself into the position of being prayed for by many people who also believe God is the power behind healing.

I believed God could heal me if He wanted, even with a "supernatural touch" as I was being prayed for. That supernatural touch was my hope and prayer. I surely didn't want the path of the operation. And I knew chemo and radiation would take a lot of "life" out of me.

However, God did not heal me through a supernatural touch as He does with some others. (See Appendix C: Stories of Supernatural Healing Today.)

I also believed He could heal me through allopathic and/or naturopathic medicine. That's why I traveled down both of those roads as well.

And I believe He is the source of healing and the ultimate cause of healing and the effectual cause of healing. In other words, ALL healing in whatever forms or means originates from Him.

Why do these healing ways come from Him?

God is The Healer for These Reasons:

1) God's kingdom operates on the reality of universal health. There is no sickness or sorrow or death in His kingdom. Anything less than that is the result of a fallen creation.

   However, since His kingdom has not fully come to earth at this point, we generally experience some health, some sickness, and ultimately death.

2) He created plants and flowers packed with nutrition and healing properties, allowing naturopathic procedures and treatments to emerge.

3) God created the physical laws of nature in the universe, allowing medical procedures and treatments to emerge because of physical law consistency.

4) He created and gifted many men and women with intellect and other abilities to develop and use all these tools for the health of the human race.

(Death is another matter. Jesus, the Good Physician is the only one who has overcome the power of death and offers eternal life.)[60]

Antioch Church Elders

So based on James 5, I called one of the elders of Antioch Church, our local church congregation in Bend, Oregon. I asked if he would set up a time with the elders after a church service when Sheri and I could be prayed for in regards to our cancer.

At this time, we knew Sheri had a return of lymphoma. So prayer for her was appropriate too.

I had some fragrant olive oil from Jerusalem which I took to the meeting. The elders gathered around us in a room, and one of them dipped his finger in the oil and put it on our foreheads in the sign of a cross. Then they placed their hands on our shoulders and each one in turn prayed for us to be healed.

Desert Streams…The Dove Network

Close friends of ours, David and Theresa Knauss,[61] attend a church in Bend where they also believe in the healing power of Jehovah Rapha.

---

[60] "Because God's children are human beings—made of flesh and blood—the Son also became flesh and blood. For only as a human being could he die, and only by dying could he break the power of the devil, who had the power of death" (Hebrews 2:14 NLT).

[61] The Knausses were colleagues working in Central Asia with us. Subsequently, they and their four children moved to Bend as well

A number of Christian leaders from their association, The Dove Network, were meeting one Saturday in the church. David invited me to come in the afternoon for prayers of healing.

Wanting to seek the Lord and do what He said, I showed up, was warmly greeted, and was ushered to a chair. Then a number of Christian leaders put their hands on my head and shoulders and prayed for my healing from the cancer in the name of Jesus and through the power of the Holy Spirit.

Bethel Church Healing Service

We had another opportunity to apply James 5 when we had the chance to attend a Saturday morning healing service in Bethel Church in Redding, California.

The pastor, Bill Johnson, is committed to seek God for healing of many sicknesses but especially to eradicate cancer in the city of Redding. His church is praying to that end.

This is a very charismatic church, and the prayer service takes place utilizing many of the gifts of the New Testament Church the Apostle Paul lists in 1 Corinthians chapter 12.

In this environment, we experienced the laying on of hands from a team of three people praying for our healing, words of wisdom pronounced over us, words of encouragement given to us, and worship songs and prayer in tongues shared throughout the time.

---

and took over as president of Life Impact Ministries, the organization we started in 2003 to care for Christian workers, (http://www.LifeImpactMinistries.net).

Sunriver Christian Fellowship

In addition to those James 5 experiences, Nancy McGrath-Green, the Episcopal priest of Sunriver Christian Fellowship, a church in Sunriver, Oregon, we were part of for eight years, came and took us through an Episcopal healing service with specific, liturgical prayers for healing.

Friends Globally Bringing Us to the Throne

And finally, I started writing my blog, www.GrissenCancerJourney.com, to keep our friends in the loop on our trials and hopeful progress with cancer. This turned into over 235 friends from all corners of the world following us on the blog and praying for us.

Each of these experiences were meaningful to us and were motivated by James 5:14-16. I guess one of my thoughts behind this was that more is better than less (as though God could be manipulated or empowered to move by my actions instead of what He already said).

What I discovered later through meditation on James 5 was that even one person praying had power with God. A group of elders certainly has influence with God as James says. But so does one righteous person.

James 5 ends with the illustration of Elijah's life regarding the rain and says, "the *prayers of one* righteous man is powerful in its effect."[62]

In order for God to be moved to action in His active will (intervening now, taking action in time and space) rather than passive will (actively choosing not to intervene, letting

---

[62] This story is found in the Old Testament in the book of 1 Kings chapter 17:1 through 18:41-48.

time and events take their course), even one righteous person offering their request will move Heaven to take action on Earth, as Elijah exemplifies.

What I did is to both seek and take advantage of many opportunities for God's people to pray for me in my battle with cancer. And to date, my testimony is the Lord has raised me up! I've had three wonderful years of life from first diagnosis.

How Do I Feel About the Fact God Didn't Supernaturally Heal Me?

I have to confess when I discovered the tumor had grown and I was not supernaturally healed by the "touch" of God on my body, I was initially disappointed. This caused me to question some of the promises on healing in the Scriptures, like James 5:14-18. Or at least to more deeply consider what they were saying and teaching.

After all, I did seek the prayers of elders—actually in four different churches as I just described. Many people prayed over me and prayed for me.

But the cancer was still there! How do I live with this? Is faith in God a mirage? Is this all a hoax? Are the atheists right that there is no God in the heavens sitting on a throne?

This also raised the question in my mind, "Does God really love ME? If so, why would He not heal me from this cancer without an operation but instead make me move forward into something I really don't want to do—a complex operation which is only 50% effective at beating down cancer at best?"

We may have different answers to that question, but after pondering this for some time, here's my answer, which satisfies my inner person (my soul). I'm sharing my thinking here in what seems accurate to me at this time.

1) God Is God. I'm Not God.

By definition, God is infinite and the ultimate person in the universe or outside of it. On the other hand, I'm a finite being, bound by time and space, created by God, and given life by His hand. I will at some point die since the unchallenged statistic is that 100% of us die.

So as much as I might like or dislike something God does, as a created being I'm in no position to challenge divinity. I simply must live with the realities He chooses for His good purposes.[63]

2) God's Thoughts Are Beyond My Thoughts.

The Bible teaches that God is omniscient—knowing everything. By contrast, I don't even know a miniscule amount of all the knowledge that exists today in the realm of human knowledge, much less divine knowledge. Can you believe it—my computer knows more than I do!

Therefore, it would be total human pride on my part to question or challenge the wisdom and thoughts of God. If He decides, for His reasons, to guide me into a medical operation rather than eradicate my cancer with a word or touch of his spiritual hand, I believe He has His reasons. Again, my responsibility is to accept whatever He chooses for me.

---

[63] "But who are you, a human being, to talk back to God? Shall what is formed say to the one who formed it, 'Why did you make me like this?'" (Romans 9:20 NLT).

And if He decides my time on Earth should end, my body will return to dust even as my spirit returns to Him. "My times are in Your hands" (Psalm 31:15).

Isaiah, the Old Testament prophet, makes a clear statement to this effect. "'My thoughts are nothing like your thoughts,' says the LORD. 'And my ways are far beyond anything you could imagine. For just as the heavens are higher than the earth, so my ways are higher than your ways and my thoughts higher than your thoughts'" Isaiah 55:8-9 (NLT).

3) God Is Not My Servant. I'm His Servant.

God has the power and authority. I do not. Therefore, He is sovereign over me. His role is to rule. My role is to serve. I am His servant, and He is not my servant.

So as much as I'd like Him to keep me healthy because He has the power to do that, as a servant I cannot make any demands on Him. (I have a personal responsibility to do all I can to preserve my health as well.)

As a loving Father, He invites me to ask for things and let Him know what I desire. But His action in regard to my request is determined in His own mind and for His own reasons. I comply with His will and not vice versa.

4) I Believe God Loves Me, so His Purposes Are Perfect for Me.

I mentioned God is revealed as a Father. It's amazing that in the Bible He is often pictured as a loving God and loving Father. Here are a couple instances to make this point:

"...yet for us there is but one God, the Father, from whom all things came and for whom we live; and there is but one Lord, Jesus Christ, through whom all things came and through whom we live" (1 Corinthians 8:6).

"See what great love the Father has lavished on us, that we should be called children of God! And that is what we are! The reason the world does not know us is that it did not know him" (1 John 3:1).

"But when you pray, go into your room, close the door and pray to your Father, who is unseen. Then your Father, who sees what is done in secret, will reward you" (Matthew 6:6).

5) Oh, Oh. Life Is Actually Like Grass or Flowers.

"As for man, his days are like grass; he flourishes like a flower of the field; the wind blows over it and it's gone, and its place remembers it no more" (Psalm 103:15-16).

"All men are like grass and all their glory is like the flowers of the field; the grass withers and the flowers fall…" (1 Peter 1:24).

From the time I was a kid growing up on a celery farm in Western Michigan until I got cancer, the idea of death was a distant mirage.

There were the older people who passed away now and then, like my Grandma who died of cancer when I was only eight years old. It was part of life for the old people to leave but not for me. We lived on, and the old people died. (Hey, now I are one!)

Even though, in the Bible life is compared to a season of grass growing, this biblical picture did not impact me in any way. After all, my dad was still living, and I figured I had years of time ahead. Life was treating me well.

Until I looked death in the face through cancer!

The first night after I knew I had cancer, I didn't sleep much. My basic question was: "Will this take me to the grave soon and shatter all my expectations of retired life?"

That night the Spirit of God (third person of the Trinity—Father, Son, and Holy Spirit) reminded me of a Bible verse, Philippians 1:25, and impressed on my mind that this truth for the Apostle Paul 2,000 years ago was also for me now: "...convinced of this [that I could still be a value to my wife, family, and friends for a time longer], I know that I will remain, and continue with all of you ..."

This took my immediate anxiety away and has proven to be true over time. I'm already in my third year from the diagnosis. (However, how much value I've been during these three years could probably be debated!)

One way this cancer journey has impacted my thinking, however, is that I now consider the brevity of life. My looming death is no longer a distant mirage. It's a present reality. How much longer do I have to live on this earth?

The end is definitely close and staring me in the face! This does cause me to consider how to order each day—by asking and answering the question, "What should I be doing today?"

6) Resurrection Proclaims: This World Is Not the End!

Personally, I don't want to die yet. How about you? I want some more years of life on this planet with Sheri, my family, and my friends. And I'm thankful I've had more days as a result of my cancer treatments.

At the same time these thoughts rattle around in my brain, I do know the stark reality: There will come a day when my life on Earth will end. And it's at this critical point where the resurrection of Jesus kicks into gear and moves us forward on all eight cylinders!

Because Jesus rose from the dead, defeated death, and gave us His promise of eternal life, I know my life does not end with my last breath from fighting cancer or something else. "For God so loved you and me that He sent His only Son, that *whoever believes* in Him will *NOT* perish, but have *ETERNAL LIFE*" (John 3:16, emphasis mine).

There is a glorious, eternal future to look forward to and live in. And according to the Bible its more glorious than anything we've experienced here on Earth, our first go-round.

Here are some glimpses into that future …

> For our light and momentary troubles are achieving for us an eternal glory that far outweighs them all (2 Corinthians 4:17 ESV).

> For I consider that the sufferings of this present time are not worth comparing with the glory that is to be revealed to us (Romans 8:18 ESV).

> He will wipe away every tear from their eyes, and death shall be no more, neither shall there be mourning, nor crying, nor pain anymore, for the former things have passed away (Revelation 21:4 ESV).

> And here is a promise given by Jesus, Himself: "In my Father's house are many rooms; if it were not so, I would have told you. I am going there to prepare a place for you. And if I go and prepare a place for you, I will come back and take you to be with me that you also may be where I am" (John 14:2-3).

In my own spiritual life I have found the Spirit of God creates a deep confidence in the heart and soul that there is an eternity out there.

A wise king once said, "Yet God has made everything beautiful for its own time. He has planted eternity in the human heart, but even so, people cannot see the whole scope of God's work from beginning to end" (Ecclesiastes 3:11).

My personal belief is in a life hereafter based on the resurrection of Jesus and His promises. So my earthly demise at some sooner rather than later point does not create anxiety in my life now. My hope is I can live out a few more years on this earth, but I'm confident something even better is waiting when my last breath is taken.

7)   There Is Suffering in This World—I Am Not Immune.

We are not living in an ideal and perfect world. All around us is so much suffering that if we meditate on it too long, we can get depressed. Many people blame God for all the problems instead of blaming ourselves. That's probably natural because He's the one who has the power to keep it from happening.

While that's true, He doesn't step in arbitrarily to stop all suffering. If He did, every human will would be overridden, and we would end up being God's robots. Instead we are God's created children who possess our own brain and can make our own decisions according to our own wills.

If God related to us as a dictator, He would be like a parent taking care of a newborn baby, determining every move for that baby. Instead, He's like a parent taking care of a teenager or young adult who makes their own decisions as they grow up.

Remember God is pictured as a good Father and not a ruling despot who determines how we should live and think and forces us that way. He allows us the privilege to think, decide, and take actions we want to take.

Therefore, in the big picture God's rulership of this world takes into account our own decisions, the actions of the devil, natural laws, and what He desires for purposes beyond our understanding.

All of these things form the mosaic of life that moves all things forward according to His secret, sovereign, active, and passive wills.

Ultimately, He prevails without forcing us to conform to His wishes. But He does so with our wills fully engaged in His decisions.

We each make our own decisions in life and must, therefore, live with the responsibility for what we decide. God will hold us accountable for our decisions in His judgment at the end of time.

We are free to blame God for anything we want. Whether that's a wise strategy for us is debatable. Certainly the Bible reveals a strong warning not to move in that direction in our relationship with the Almighty. Obedience to Him is the value rather than rebellion.

So my understanding is God does not create suffering. Nor does He step in each and every time to stop it. Therefore, since the world is full of suffering created by:

- nature in turmoil,
- governmental powers,
- decisions of other human beings that negatively affect me,
- my own bad decisions

why should I think I could be exempt from suffering in my life?

Even if I was a perfect man and made no bad decisions myself, I would still be subject to the other factors that create suffering.

So at a very basic level, my cancer is a result of living in this world and experiencing the negative results of nature (dis-ease). It is not the direct result of God shafting me in some way. He is only sending love my way.

The Benefits of Suffering

The fact is, suffering is an existential reality for each of us. None of us is immune or escapes from various types of suffering as we live our lives.

How we deal with this reality when it blasts into our lives is the issue. Faith in Jesus reveals that suffering, while a difficult element for any of us to face and manage, does have redeeming value in the big scheme of things.

In other words, there are positives to gain from this significant negative. Or we could say in "eclipse language," the sun in our lives will return as the darkness passes out of range.

The Bible teaches that God gives a perspective on suffering that helps us carry it instead of being immobilized or embittered by it.

Armed with this perspective and the power He puts into our lives through His Spirit, we are in a great position to take advantage of the benefits of suffering.

Here are some statements from the Bible regarding the benefits we gain from suffering:

Benefit 1: Development of Our Character

"Not only so, but we also glory in our sufferings, because we know that suffering produces perseverance;

perseverance, character; and character, hope."
(Romans 5:3-4)

And…

"Count it all joy, my brothers, when you meet trials of various kinds, for you know that the testing of your faith produces steadfastness. And let steadfastness have its full effect, that you may be perfect and complete, lacking in nothing" (James 1:2-3 ESV).

Benefit 2: Deepening of Our Spiritual Life

"He humbled you, causing you to hunger and then feeding you with manna, which neither you nor your ancestors had known, to teach you that man does not live on bread alone but on every word that comes from the mouth of the Lord" (Deuteronomy 8:3).

Benefit 3: Gaining Inner Strength to Stop Doing the Bad Things We Do

"Therefore, since Christ suffered in His body, arm yourselves with the same resolve, because anyone who has suffered in his body is done with sin. Consequently, he does not live out his remaining time on earth for human passions, but for the will of God" (1 Peter 4:1 Berean Study Bible).

Peter indicates that suffering creates within us the inner condition of 'being done with sin.' In other words, we are enabled to overcome our passions and evil desires, and do what's good and right in God's sight. This is a powerful result of our suffering.

Benefit 4: Experiencing God in the Midst of Suffering

"The righteous person may have many troubles, but the Lord delivers him from them all" (Psalm 34:17).

As we see in my case, this 'deliverance' doesn't always come as we might wish. But in the process of trusting God for deliverance, we do experience Him in ways that build us up as people.

<u>Benefit 5: Making Us Stronger as a Person</u>

"And after you have suffered a little while, the God of all grace, who has called you to his eternal glory in Christ, will himself restore, confirm, strengthen, and establish you" (1 Peter 5:10 ESV).

<u>Benefit 6: Having the Inner Confidence My Suffering</u>
<u>Works for My Good</u>

"And we know that for those who love God all things [including suffering] work together for good, for those who are called according to his purpose"
(Romans 8:28 ESV).

The Bible is quite clear—suffering can't be escaped, but there is a silver lining in it for those trusting God when they are suffering. Spiritual benefits are conferred on the sufferer which enriches their life. We are winners when it appears we are loser.

What Happens if the Cancer Returns?

This is a scary question—one I'd rather not think about. However, the only option to not thinking about this is to go into denial. It is a question always on the horizon.

My oncologist suggested with the operation, I might "hit a home run," and it would be gone. One of my naturopaths said, "Cancer is never gone. You must keep fighting."

So I've decided to live as though I hit a home run and eat and exercise like the cancer could come back.

Perhaps that's a little "schizophrenic." But the challenge is in how I'm thinking about it. I want to believe the cancer is gone and I'm healed. That's the medical case, and the health of my body backs that up.

That's how I also feel about the spiritual case. I believe that through all I've been through in the last three years and how I've come out, God has healed me.

Yet with any little change in swallowing or body function, my mind goes immediately to the fear that cancer has returned.

For example, one day I felt a hard lump in the side of my throat. This seemed to be a lymph gland, and my immediate thought was "Cancer is in my lymph system now."

This is not a far-fetched conclusion given my whole situation. Fortunately, the next day the gland seemed soft and normal again; so the fear dissipated.

The day after that it was hard again, and the fear returned. The next day it was gone. Relief. I felt like I was on a rollercoaster. What was happening?

As it turns out, I'd had a hernia operation at that time, and the anesthesia for the operation was working itself out of the body through my lymph system. So I happened to feel the gland both times at the time it was working overtime to process those chemicals.

I discovered this fact by googling "lymph nodes." Dr. Martin, my oncologist, confirmed this when I saw him a week later. I've not had a return of this phenomenon since.

So this is one of my emotional after-effects of the cancer eclipse. I'll have to live with it and process as it happens.

Treatment Options If Cancer Returns

1) <u>Allopathic Options</u>: If cancer returns, it would undoubtedly be metastasized, in which case the only medical option would be chemo to try and control it for a palliative care.

   It is also possible that by that time research may have discovered some other option which could work, such as immunotherapy. Today medical knowledge is multiplying rapidly, at the blink of an eye.

2) <u>Naturopathic Options</u>: If the cancer does return, I could also go the naturopathic route with additional treatments again. When Roy Bennett found out he had Stage IV esophageal cancer he decided to go with natural treatments. That's when he discovered the CIPAG Clinic in Mexico, had treatments, and lived another seven years before passing away August 1, 2017. (See his story in Appendix A: Four Stories of Other Esophageal Cancer Warriors.)

3) <u>Anointing and Prayer Again</u>: And finally, if I sensed the return of cancer was not "supposed to take me to my end," I would again call the elders of my church to anoint me with oil and pray for me to be healed based on James 5:14-18. If I sensed, however, that this was now my end, I would prepare myself for the passage into eternity.

FORWARD...ONWARD . . .

Thanks for reading the unfolding, three-year story of my cancer eclipse. Fortunately its not the "never ending story!" Why not?

Because as this book was going to print I had my first CT scan after my operation. That was an eight-month time gap. Dr. Martin came into the room with the results and said, "The scans are great. Your cancer is gone. You are cancer free!"

Now we know twenty soldiers were defeated! Now the sun is shining again in my life, as it is for Sheri.

It's a deep and satisfying relief to have this behind us although ongoing doctor visits to monitor progress are still on the calendar. Those are normally short and encouraging, pushing us forward with life and health.

If you are entering the cancer eclipse or are still in it, we want to join hands with you as we can. Please connect with us, and if you desire prayer for your situation, please let us know that as well. (CancerEclipse@gmail.com)

If you already came through a cancer eclipse yourself, we are thankful for that reality with you. Send us a short note to give us a glimpse of your path. Those notes will encourage us as well.

We don't know how you are, or will, process your post-cancer life. For us cancer relief raised an important question we wrestle with: *"What should be our purpose of life going forward in the final days we have left?"*

Our religious background in the Reformed Church of America introduced us to the Westminster Catechism, approved by the Church of Scotland in 1640.

This document concisely spells out in question-answer form the belief system of the Reformed and Presbyterian churches. Those churches emerged out of the Protestant Reformation in 1517, led by Martin Luther.

One question in the catechism raises the same issue I mentioned above, but in a different form: *"What is the chief and highest end of man?"*

The answer of this old document, drafted almost 450 years ago, is still helpful and instructive: *"Man's chief and highest end is to glorify God and fully to enjoy him forever."*

While this answer does not fill in the daily details of how we can expend our lives post-cancer, it does give us an overarching direction for that pursuit.

And at the same time, it answers one of the four major elements of our worldview: *"Why are we here?"*

If I understand this correctly, the focus of our lives going forward and onward in the days we have left should not be absorbed with ourselves.

First, we should ensure God is the focal point and relational enjoyment of our lives. And secondly, we should ensure we make a positive difference in the lives of people around us.

Getting past the self-absorption is the big challenge. But worship and service, it seems, could help us get there.

Then with this overarching direction guiding us, our remaining time on this planet can still be invested wisely. And the result will be a positive impact in our world because we lived here.

May the Sun, and the Son, keep shining on all of us!

APPENDIX A

Four Stories of Other Esophageal Cancer Warriors

As I fought esophageal cancer, I connected with a few others who experienced a cancer eclipse and who have their own stories of the fight against this type of cancer. I thought you'd be interested to read a few short synopses of telephone interviews I had with them. (Roy's story was taken from the CIPAG website).

Beating the Statistics at Stage IV[64]

Roy Bennet

British Columbia, CANADA

After having difficulty swallowing in August 2010, I went to my doctor and was eventually diagnosed in October 2010, with Stage IV esophageal cancer.

---

[64] (www.drcastillo.com).

My doctor explained this was a very aggressive cancer and immediately arranged for consultations with a radiologist, oncologist, and surgeon.

The radiologist wanted to start radiation ASAP to try and reduce the size of the cancer so the surgeon could remove it. The surgery would be followed by chemotherapy.

I met with the surgeon, and he explained that due to the location and type of cancer, he would remove my entire esophagus and move my stomach up into my throat area (esophagectomy). He told me recovery to a semi-normal lifestyle would take about eighteen months, and there was a reasonable probability that the cancer would return somewhere else.

For many years I had taught divine healing at my church, and I felt that if I really believed God still heals, then it was time to put my faith in to action.

I refused any radiation treatment and told both my doctor and surgeon that I was not going to have treatments. My doctor told me that I would eventually starve to death and asked if I would sign a form giving him permission to insert a feeding tube when the time came.

The surgeon was quite upset at my decision and told me that unless I had the operation, I would be back in three months, and he would only be able to offer me palliative care.

[Note: If my understanding of stages is correct (see Chapter 1), I think Roy was looking at metastasis and palliative care from the outset unless staging is different in

Canada. And he does mention that when diagnosed, his doctor gave him three months to live without treatment.]

I appreciate they were advising me to do what they felt was best for me, but I made my decision to trust God for my healing.

Shortly after this, a friend came to our home with a bag of vegetables and a DVD. She told me to juice the vegetables and watch the video. I did what she told me. The video, which described alternative cancer treatments, started my wife searching for these ways of alternative medical care.

In that search, we came across the webpage for the Castillo Clinic, CIPAG, and read the testimonies. Then I placed a call to Dr. Castillo in Tijuana, Mexico. [See Chapter 6 for more on CIPAG.]

He called me back later that day. In the conversation we discussed my condition, and Dr. Castillo told me to come down to the clinic as soon as possible.

My wife and I arrived at the clinic in January of 2011. We were impressed with the friendliness of the staff, especially Dr. Castillo, who is a very caring, compassionate man, genuinely committed to helping his patients.

He spent a lot of time explaining my condition, the treatment program he recommended, and what he felt they could accomplish for me. I found him to be a "straight shooter" who did not sugarcoat my situation.

As I started my treatment, I met so many people who had amazing stories about the clinic and the success of patients with almost every kind of sickness or disease.

A large number of them had been given short-term terminal diagnoses by their doctors but many years later were doing well and, in some cases, were totally healed and cancer-free.

I cannot say enough about my experience at the clinic. I would recommend to anyone who has any kind of disease or sickness to call Dr. Castillo and discuss their condition with him.

I believe that God directed me to the clinic because our bodies have amazing abilities to heal themselves if we just take care of them. With the help of Dr. Castillo and his staff I am in better shape than I have ever been in my life.

I will continue to receive treatments and look to God to complete my healing.

Because of my advanced stage of esophageal cancer, the doctors gave me three months to live when my cancer was discovered. I should have already been dead in early 2011. Instead I am now one of those people at the clinic who can testify and encourage others as they arrive for the first time.

[Note: Roy's testimony given above was taken from the CIPAG Clinic website. I talked with Roy via phone about the Castillo Clinic on August 12, 2016, regarding my own situation.

He was doing great then. (In fact, he had just come back into the house after a 4-wheeler ride on his property.) But he said he felt the tumor may be growing a little. The tip-off to growth was his swallowing getting a little harder. He said he should probably see Dr. Castillo again.

On September 7, 2017, I called him again to see how he was doing. His wife answered the phone and said Roy had passed away on August 1, 2017. The esophageal cancer had metastasized into his liver.

He was seventy-four years old when he passed away but had seven more years of quality of life from the time of his original diagnosis to his death.

Roy beat the statistics without the chemo-radiation-operation protocol, using natural means and trusting the healing hand of God for extended life! And he did that with the tumor still in his body. Unfortunately, it was finally the cause of his death.]

Beating the Medical Protocol at Stage IV

Bob Haase[65]

Hubbard Lake, Michigan

I was diagnosed with Stage IV esophageal cancer in 2010 because the cancer had spread to my lymph nodes. To remedy the situation, I had eighteen weeks of chemo treatments that successfully cleared the cancer at that time.

However, in 2012, the cancer reappeared in the esophagus.

---

[65] Bob is willing to discuss his situation with anyone interested in learning more. Call him at (989) 727-2793.

I then underwent five weeks of radiation treatments (intensity-modulated radiation therapy), and again the cancer was cleared in the esophagus.

But a year later in 2013, it appeared once more in my esophagus.

At that time, the choice my oncologist gave me was chemo for palliative care (as a last resort) or the esophagectomy. However, the thoracic surgeons at the University of Michigan were unwilling to do this surgery because my cancer was Stage IV and had already metastasized beyond the tumor site.

My oncologist then set up an appointment for me at the Cleveland Clinic with the Thoracic Surgery Department. After consulting with them, they referred me to the Gastroenterology Department with Dr. Sunguk Jang.

Dr. Jang was willing to do the operation and successfully removed the tumor from the lower esophagus via endoscopic mucosal resection. Once the cancer was removed he treated me five times using radio frequency ablation[66] to remove the

---

[66] According to Cancer Centers of America, needle-based ablation is a localized treatment using high-energy radio waves to heat and destroy cancerous cells. During this procedure, a thin, needle-like probe is temporarily inserted into a tumor through a tiny incision in the skin, using CT scan or ultrasound guidance. The probe then releases electrodes that heat and destroy cancer cells. This procedure is delivered by microwave technology or via needle-based implementation. This is used when surgery is not an option or to relieve other symptoms, (https://www.cancercenter.com/treatments/needle-based-ablation/).

Barrett's condition in the lower esophagus, which was the source of the cancer.

These procedures utilize the endoscopic equipment with very little after effects. Subsequent scans and endoscopic exams have shown no reoccurring cancer or Barrett's.

I would encourage some esophageal cancer patients like me to investigate alternatives to the major surgery being considered. I was very satisfied with the Cleveland Clinic Doctors and particularly Dr. Sunguk Jang. His staff information is on this site, https://my.clevelandclinic.org/staff/7662-sunguk-jang. For an appointment call (216) 444-7000.

I still have follow-up procedures with my local oncologist and normally do a yearly endoscopic exam and a CT scan to track the existence of cancer. At this point there is no recurrence of Barrett's condition or the tumors.

My one lingering side effect has been acid reflux, particularly at night when I sleep. To control this, I was taking TUMS. However, now my oncologist has prescribed a daily, 40mg tablet dose of Pantoprazole Sod to ward off any acid reflux.

This has worked and stopped the occurrence of acid reflux. And according to the manufacturer, Pantoprazole SOD also helps heal acid damage to the stomach and esophagus, helps prevent ulcers, and may help prevent cancer of the esophagus.

Beating Cancer & Depression Afterwards

Don Moore[67]

Holland, Michigan

At age seventy-one, in 2010, I was having a swallowing issue. So I went to my general doctor, and he immediately suspected cancer. I ended up with a Barium test and CT scan.

The results came back with a diagnosis of esophageal cancer and a 35% survival rating IF I would have the standard protocol: chemo-radiation-esophagectomy.

Because I didn't have medical insurance but rather Medicare, I chose to utilize the Veteran's Administration Hospital in Ann Arbor, Michigan, since I am a vet and also a resident of Zeeland, Michigan.

The doctors at the VA told me their survival rate for the esophagectomy was higher than the national average because of the type of patient they'll do operations for. They will not take someone who's obese or has other health issues. If the vet who wants the operation is not in good shape, they will not do the esophagectomy for them.

I was in good shape but was also a smoker. They told me to stop smoking for six weeks, or they wouldn't do the operation. I stopped smoking.

---

[67] Don is willing to discuss his situation with anyone interested in learning more. Call him at (616) 399-1871.

I was questioning whether to have the operation or not, but they told me my cancer would probably come back within two years if I didn't have the esophagectomy. Therefore, I made the decision to have it.

My operation lasted nine hours, and then I was in hospital recovery for two more weeks. Finally, I was released into a rehabilitation home in Holland, Michigan, for another month.

One unfortunate event happened to me in rehab. I was given morphine to control my pain. I didn't realize I was allergic to morphine, but the drug makes me depressed. So I went into a deep depression in the rehab center, without knowing the problem. After the month, I left in that depression.

A psychiatrist helped me through this difficult time of weaning myself off morphine and working through all the issues the operation and the allergic reaction had created.

While in rehab, my appetite was also negligible, so I had to continue on my feeding tube. I was finished with the tube by the time I left rehab and eating small portions of normal food five or six times a day.

Because of the operation, rehab, and recovery, I lost 100 pounds which brought me down to a healthier weight of around 198 pounds. After all these years I am now at a point where I can gain weight again through eating, although I don't need to.

I was told by the doctors the esophagectomy was more difficult than a heart transplant. My wife said it took me six months to get to my new "normal."

Since my operation, I've had CT scans every six months for a couple years, but now I have one annually. I am six years out from my operation and therefore in the 50% of survivors making it longer than that period of time.

Here's what Don shared was his new "normal:"

- Eating about one-third of his former normal meal at mealtimes. (Eating the smaller portions creates a normal intestinal system function.)

- Eating more often per day than he did before.

- Sitting up two hours after he eats to control the acid reflux.

- Eating too much at one time causes vomiting. (Knowing when he is full of food only happens when the amount reaches throat level.)

- To control acid reflux without his hiatal valve, he takes more TUMS than the average person.

Don's recommendation for esophagectomy patients:

The esophagectomy takes a lot of energy out of a person, so being or getting into good physical health prior to having it is vital. This is an important issue in his view.

[Note: I would add, build up your immune system via natural methods, supplements, and healthy food prior to having the esophagectomy so your body is strong going into treatment.]

Beating Cancer for the Long Haul

John Jankuski[68]

Atlanta, Georgia

In 1996, when I was fifty-six years old, I was diagnosed with esophageal cancer and had a large tumor. I don't remember what my stage was, but I don't think my lymph glands were affected.

[Note: He had a tremendously hard chemo both before and after so perhaps they were.]

I had chemo-radiation for six weeks and upon reflection think it might have been overkill. After these treatments were completed, it took me two months to recover. Then I went in for my esophagectomy. The operation was successful because I've been cancer free for eighteen years.

Here is my advice for those going through this:

- Keep up your attitude—stay positive.

- Stay in good physical condition—I believe this helped me come through it well.

- Don't let friends or family determine what you do. I had friends who had the operation in Atlanta, whereas I went to Johns Hopkins because I felt that was the best center for me. All but one of my friends is dead. You have to go with your own instincts.

---

[68] John is willing to discuss his situation with anyone interested in learning more. Call him at (770) 231-5734.

- Don't worry about traveling to another location. Get the best medical help you can find anywhere. It's your life on the line.

- The operation was worth doing—this is a BAD cancer!

Here's a summary of what my operation entailed:

- I was nauseous throughout the whole process— chemo-radiation as well as post-surgery.

- I had two months to recover from radiation-chemo, and then I went into surgery.

- The chemo-radiation had shrunk the tumor to almost nothing. I then went ahead with the operation for two reasons: First, I was in a medical study and needed to proceed. Second, I wanted to get rid of the tumor—get it out of my body. That was my attitude.

- It took at least a year from start to finish before I was back to normal. After eighteen months I was back to normal work as a pilot. I got my pilot's license back and finished up my career for three years. I retired at age sixty.

- My operation was in July. In January the following year I went in for three shots of chemo again. These were also difficult for my body.

- During my chemo-radiation I stayed in the Hackemas-Patch House on the campus of Johns-Hopkins for one month. During surgery I was in the hospital for ten days, and my wife stayed in the house. Of those ten days, four of them were in the intensive care unit.

- I wanted to get back home quickly. So shortly after I was released from the hospital I left and went back to Atlanta via airplane. That was a tough trip because I left too soon.

My Quality of Life after the Esophagectomy:

- Initially I had pain when eating and would double-over from the pain.

- My food took a "free fall," all the way to the colon.

- I had difficulty eating initially. Now I eat everything I want without problems, even Mexican food and other very spicy foods.

- I eat smaller portions, however, and I've learned how much I can have at a time.

- I also eat several times more each day, but remember, "That's healthy, right?"

- I feel uncomfortable if I get too much food. Food then backs up, and I feel it. If I get too much, I still have to vomit it up.

- I never lost my ability to swallow, nor do I have any problems swallowing now.

- My BIGGEST after-effect came from radiation. It affected my heart fifteen years later at age seventy-one. This side effect gave me an atrial flutter (not A-fib). I now have a pacemaker, but I don't feel it or think about it much.

[Note: This is one of the potential side effects from the operation that was mentioned to me. In my last checkup, my oncologist thought I might have it. I had an EKG and was thankful my test proved negative for A-fib.]

APPENDIX B[69]

You're Kidding! Coffee Enemas from Max Gerson?

(Release by the Gerson Institute)

We would like to briefly reiterate the purpose of coffee enemas because many people new to the therapy ask about this. Also, this is a reminder to enema "veterans" for how we can explain this to others.

Coffee enemas are a vital part of the detoxification process of the Gerson Therapy. The purpose of the enemas is to remove toxins accumulated in the liver and to remove free radicals from the bloodstream.

In the 1920s, two German professors tested the effects of infused caffeine on rats. They found that the caffeine travels via the hemorrhoidal vein and the portal system to the liver, opens up the bile ducts and allows the liver to release bile, which contains toxins. The theobromine, theophylline, and the caffeine in coffee dilate blood vessels and bile ducts, relax smooth muscles, and increase the bile flow.

---

[69] The information regarding the coffee enemas and bio of Dr. Max Gerson is taken from the Gerson Institute website, (https://gerson.org/gerpress/dr-max-gerson/).

Doctors at the University of Minnesota showed that coffee administered rectally also stimulates an enzyme system in the liver called glutathione S-transferase by 600%-700% above normal activity levels. This enzyme reacts with free radicals (which cause cell damage) in the bloodstream and makes them inert.

These neutralized substances become dissolved in the bile, are released through the bile flow from the liver and gallbladder, and are excreted through the intestinal tract.

A Gerson patient holds the coffee enema in the colon for 12-15 minutes. During this time, the body's entire blood supply passes through the liver 4-5 times, carrying poisons picked up from the tissues. So the enema acts as a form of dialysis of the blood across the gut wall.

The purpose of the coffee enema is not to clear out the intestines, but the quart of water in the enema stimulates peristalsis in the gut. A portion of the water also dilutes the bile and increases the bile flow, thereby flushing toxic bile (loaded with toxins by the glutathione S-transferase enzyme system) out of the intestines.

A patient coping with a chronic degenerative disease or an acute illness can achieve the following benefits from the lowering of blood serum toxin levels achieved by regular administration of coffee enemas:

1) increased cell energy production
2) enhanced tissue health
3) improved blood circulation
4) better immunity and tissue repair, and
5) cellular regeneration

Additionally, coffee enemas can help to relieve pain, nausea, general nervous tension and depression.

References: "A Cancer Therapy: Results of Fifty Cases" by Dr. Gerson, "Healing the Gerson Way" by Charlotte Gerson, and "Liver Detoxification with Coffee Enemas" by Morton Walker, DPM excerpted from July 2001 edition of Townsend Newsletter, Phone (619) 685-5353, info@gerson.org www.gerson.org.

Dr. Max Gerson

Max Gerson, MD, was born in Wongrowitz, Germany (1881). He attended the universities of Breslau, Wurzburg, Berlin, and Freiburg. Suffering from severe migraines, Dr. Gerson focused his initial experimentation with diet on preventing his headaches.

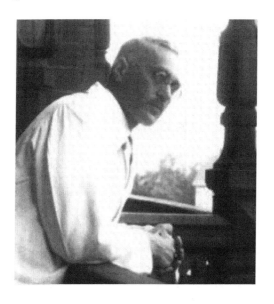

One of Dr. Gerson's patients discovered in the course of his treatment that the "migraine diet" had cured his skin tuberculosis. This discovery led Gerson to further study the diet, and he went on to successfully treat many tuberculosis patients.

His work eventually came to the attention of famed thoracic surgeon, Ferdinand Sauerbruch, MD. Under Sauerbruch's supervision, Dr. Gerson established a special skin tuberculosis treatment program at the Munich University Hospital.

In a carefully monitored clinical trial, 446 out of 450 skin tuberculosis patients treated with the Gerson diet recovered completely. Dr. Sauerbruch and Dr. Gerson simultaneously published articles in a dozen of the world's leading medical journals, establishing the Gerson treatment as the first cure for skin tuberculosis.

At this time, Dr. Gerson attracted the friendship of Nobel prize winner Albert Schweitzer, MD, by curing Schweitzer's wife of lung tuberculosis after all conventional treatments had failed. Gerson and Schweitzer remained friends for life and maintained regular correspondence.

Dr. Schweitzer followed Gerson's progress as the dietary therapy was successfully applied to heart disease, kidney failure, and finally — cancer. Schweitzer's own type II diabetes was cured by treatment with Gerson's therapy.

In 1938, Dr. Gerson passed his boards and was licensed to practice in the state of New York. For twenty years, he treated hundreds of cancer patients who had been given up to die after all conventional treatments had failed.

A Cancer Therapy: Results of 50 Cases

In 1946, Gerson brought recovered patients before the Pepper-Neely Congressional Subcommittee during hearings on a bill to fund research into cancer treatment. Although only a few peer-reviewed journals were receptive to Gerson's then "radical" idea that diet could affect health, he continued to publish articles on his therapy and case histories of healed patients.

In 1958, after thirty years of clinical experimentation, Gerson published *A Cancer Therapy: Results of 50 Cases*. This medical monograph details the theories, treatment, and results achieved by this exceptional physician.

Gerson died in 1959, eulogized by long-time friend, Albert Schweitzer MD:

> ...I see in him one of the most eminent geniuses in the history of medicine. Many of his basic ideas have been adopted without having his name connected with them. Yet, he has achieved more than seemed possible under adverse conditions. He leaves a legacy which commands attention and which will assure him his due place. Those whom he has cured will now attest to the truth of his ideas.[70]

Dr. Max Gerson: Healing the Hopeless

You can read the full story of Dr. Max Gerson's life and the development of the Gerson Therapy in his biography, *Dr. Max Gerson: Healing the Hopeless*, written by his grandson, Howard Straus.

Dr. Max Gerson: Healing the Hopeless discusses the development of his world-famous dietary therapy and the struggles this medical pioneer faced as he challenged orthodox medicine with his nutritional protocol.

This inspiring and uplifting biography follows Dr. Gerson through Nazi persecution; persecution in the United States from the medical establishment; the continuation of

---

[70] Quote by Albert Schweitzer found on the Gerson website, (https://gerson.org/gerpress/dr-max-gerson/).

his work despite the opposition; his questionable death; his daughter Charlotte's work; and finally, the present, where the Gerson Institute works to continue his legacy and vision.

[Note: When you purchase this book via the URL below, you will be supporting the organization Sheri and I started, Life Impact Ministries, which strengthens international Christian workers and pastors.]

(https://smile.amazon.com/Dr-Max-Gerson-Healing Hopeless/dp/0976018616/ref=sr_1_1?ie=UTF8&qid=1507209 704&sr=81&keywords=dr+max+gerson+healing+the+hopel ess)

APPENDIX C

Stories of Supernatural Healing Today

God is involved with our healing today by various means—allopathic and naturopathic medicine, the healing power of our bodies, and His supernatural touch.

As you saw, my story has much to do with all of these ways of healing.

However, one question that comes up with any discussion of supernatural healing is why we don't see more of it in our culture.

I believe there are more supernatural healings out there than we realize. We are just not looking in the right places, or connected to those who are seeing more of that happening. Happening today it is, however.

So I'm offering you a few stories where God moved in His sovereignly and healed someone without all the means we normally attribute to healing.

These are credible stories because we know the personal integrity of these friends. And one of these comes out of our own experience with our oldest son.

Born Breach with a Broken Shoulder

Troy Grissen, our son

We didn't realize the implications when the doctor told us our oldest son, Troy, would be born breach.

However, in 1972, when he finally came into this world feet first, it was a difficult birth for him, and Sheri suffered from it as well.

The nerves on one arm and shoulder were stretched leaving his arm useless by his side. His collarbone was broken on the other. Our dear son lay in his crib with a sling on his broken arm, unable to raise either arm.

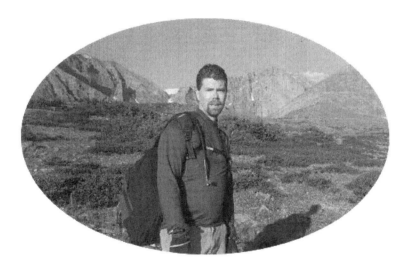

Of course, we prayed for him, as did others, and were hoping the Lord would somehow act to heal his arms. Eventually the sling came off, but he still did not have much motion with either arm.

Then I thought about the Apostle Paul and his experience with the "thorn in his flesh" documented in 2

Corinthians 12:8-9. "Three times I pleaded with the Lord to take it away from me. But he said to me, 'My grace is sufficient for you, for my power is made perfect in weakness.' Therefore, I will boast all the more gladly about my weaknesses, so that Christ's power may rest on me."

I thought, "Based on this experience, I can at least ask the Lord three times to heal my son." So I asked once in a special prayer. A few weeks later when nothing had happened to his arm movement, I asked again.

He was born on July 6, 1972, and it was now September 4, 1972, the day of our fourth wedding anniversary. Sheri and I were planning to go out for a celebration dinner and were dressing for the occasion. Troy was lying quietly on our bed—our next task was to get him ready for the babysitter.

Suddenly out of the corner of my eye I caught some motion. Looking at my son lying on the bed, I hollered to Sheri, "Look at this. Quick!"

Troy was laying there with both arms moving simultaneously over his head—the first time in his life that had happened. What an anniversary present for us and what a growth blessing for his physical body.

His arms have not bothered him since then. He's gone on to live a normal life: play basketball, soccer, and go cycling, renovate houses, and be a mechanical engineer with the full use of both of his arms.

And he's lifted his own children in his arms as well! A blessing of healing in 1972, a blessing of quality of life for our son, and a blessing for us as his parents! Thank you, Jehovah Rapha!

Supernatural Healing of a Leper—in the 21st Century?

Soar, Citizen of Mozambique

Here's a story that encouraged us from a missionary friend of ours, Brenda Lange, who works with orphans and establishing new churches in Mozambique. (www.OrphansUnlimited.org)

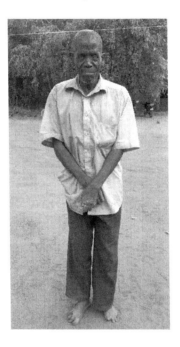

Soar (So-R), a leper, was abandoned by his family because of his illness. He received hospital treatment for his leprosy last year but still lost fingers and toes. For unknown reasons he became bedridden for many months. Surviving with the help of a few villagers, he somehow heard people talk about Jesus, the Healer.

He sent a messenger to ask the church members in his village to come to his hut to pray for him because his leprosy prevented him from walking.

When they prayed with and for him, he repented of his sins and asked Jesus to save him.

Nothing happened immediately, but over the next few weeks his faith in Jesus grew as he kept thanking Jesus for his healing. He soon regained strength in his legs and began walking short distances.

Last Sunday he surprised the Nacala Church members by WALKING into the Sunday service, demanding to tell them what Jesus had done in his life!

November 30 was salary day and our monthly meeting for all our "Bush Pastors". When Soar heard of this meeting, he asked Pastor Salazar if he could walk with him to give his testimony to ALL our pastors. That meant a 7 kilometer (3.8 mile) walk!

Salazar told me he was doubtful Soar's legs would hold, but Soar wanted to tell everyone what Jesus did for him.

He Made It to the Meeting!

Tired but happy, Soar shared his story, leaving not a dry eye in the group, for he displayed such humility as he told his story.

At the end, our church gifted him with money to buy new clothes because he only had the clothes he was wearing.

He begged me to take back the money and give him food instead, for he had little to eat at his mud hut.

Through an interpreter of his tribal dialect, I told him to buy new clothes and that Jesus would also gift him with food each month.

He walked away with a smile on his face and a week's worth of food in a sack hung over his shoulder.

Such are the reality and the values of the Kingdom of God!

Why Was the Namara Church Filled to Overflowing Today?

Here's another story from Brenda Lange's work among orphans in Mozambique. This story demonstrates further that supernatural healings are happening in our world today through prayer in the powerful name of Jesus. "For there is no other name under heaven, given among men, by which we must be saved!" (Acts 4:12).

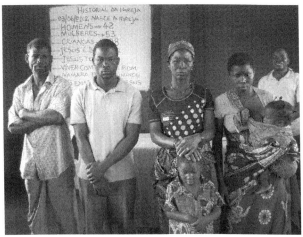

l to r: Laurinda's husband, Armindo, Laurinda & son,
Armindo's wife & Alishandrina

Armindo, twenty years old, and his daughter, Alishandrina, two years old, had been sick for over three months. Armindo had a swollen leg from an abscess that wouldn't heal, and his daughter was ill with constant stomach pain.

Armindo's Muslim mother, Laurinda, took them both to the witchdoctor and the local mosque for healing multiple times but without success.

Then Laurinda heard about Jesus' healing power.

In the middle of the night, when no one was around, she took her son and granddaughter to our church building in the Namara village. As they knelt on the floor, she asked this "Jesus" to heal her children.

Instantly, the baby's stomach pain stopped, Arminda's leg swelling disappeared, and the abscess healed over. I saw his leg this morning, and all that was visible was some peeling skin where the abscess had been. The two year old was sleeping peacefully in her mother's arms.

Pastor Ramadane of Namara knew nothing of this until Laurinda came to his house last Saturday. She asked permission to tell her story in church the next day.

Today, I (Brenda) met the entire family. All four of them realize Jesus is the Messiah and have given their allegiance to Him as the true God.

Following a Chicken Leads to Healings in Indonesia

Here is another amazing story of God's divine healing in our world today. This incident is documented in the book *Amazing Modern Day Miracles*[71], by Suzanne Frey, and shared in my blog post with her permission.

One day, my friends Julie and Moush and I were on an outreach trip in Surabaya, Indonesia, and had a few hours to spare. Desiring that God would move powerfully through us with His compassion and love, we went to Surabaya's main village store and bought a lot of food and candy and then asked God for a clue as to where to go.

Now the Holy Spirit speaks in both creative and mysterious ways. As we were praying for direction about the "who" He wanted us to share His love with, we felt God bring to our minds the word "chicken."

"What did that mean?" we asked ourselves. We continued walking through the streets of Surabaya, asking God to show us where He wanted us to go.

---

[71] Note: If you want to purchase this book, use the URL below. At the same time you purchase this book, you'll be supporting Life Impact Ministries (www.LifeImpactMinistries.net), the organization Sheri and I started to care for Christian workers. (https://smile.amazon.com/Amazing-Modern-Day-Miracles-Stories-Strengthen/dp/0736965688/ref=sr_1_1?ie=UTF8&qid=1507230898&sr=8-1&keywords=Suzanne+Frey).

Suddenly, we saw a chicken walking down the sidewalk.

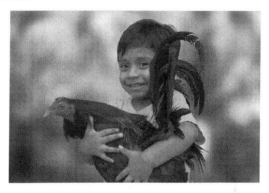

With our bags of candy and food in hand, the three of us started following the chicken as it walked along. The chicken turned into a dark alley. So we followed it down there. When we came out on the other side of the alley, we found ourselves in the courtyard of a small Muslim *kampung* neighborhood, which is similar to a slum.

We entered the *kampung*, where twenty children and their parents came out to the courtyard to meet us. We started giving them the food and candy we'd bought.

No one in the *kampung* spoke English. Yet we found a way to communicate and ask if anyone had any sickness or injuries we could pray for so they could be healed.

An old lady came forward. Sitting in a chair in front of us, she looked at us and pointed to her knees and then to a spot on her back. Believing God wanted to move in compassion and love toward her, we began praying for her.

After a short, minute-long prayer, the woman stood up and began jumping around. Jesus had completely healed her knees and back! She hugged and kissed me on the cheek and for the next hour was jumping up and down with much joy.

Right after that healing, five more ladies with similar knee and back injuries lined up for prayer. As our team prayed, we saw God touch and heal each of their injuries.

The neighborhood life erupted, and the ladies started taking us to others in the *kampung* who needed prayer for healing. A few men had shoulder and arm injuries from hard work. Jesus touched and healed every man's injury.

Heaven invaded this neighborhood; it was as if the pages from the book of Acts had come alive in this little *kampung* in Indonesia.

Does God Heal Anyone in Atlanta, Georgia?

Jehovah Rapha, the healing God, is healing in our world today in many and various ways, as He has been throughout human history. I like to document credible "supernatural touch" healing stories, and here's another one from friends of ours.

Tom and Bonnie Kopp are missionaries with Paraclete (www.Paraclete.net), training Christian leaders around the globe. They recently moved into a home in the Atlanta suburbs and had many housing issues.

Then they discovered the house had been a center for occult activity. Here's their amazing incident from the time they were moving into this home…

Just a quick note before we leave for South Africa. I know this will encourage you. We have experienced a miracle! It is difficult to explain in just a short email, but I will try.

If you recall, we had multiple problems since moving into this home which we believe have been connected to the previous owner's "meditation center" and occult objects found on the property.

Well, two weeks ago a very suspicious melanoma-looking mole appeared on the top of Tom's head. I saw it when I was cutting his hair, which I cut monthly, so I knew it was a new mole.

Our daughter, who's had three melanomas, came over and looked at the mole. She also thought it looked serious; so I made an appointment to have it checked on the Monday after Easter.

The Wednesday before Easter, at the women's Bible study I mentioned Tom's mole and that we were concerned about him having an open wound on his head during our travels in Africa, which were coming up soon.

Immediately a friend suggested they all gather around me and pray. I sat in a chair in the middle of the group, and they prayed for Tom and me.

Then on the Saturday before Easter, we were looking out the window at the "meditation circle," and Tom said, "I believe we need to remove the fountain that is in the center of that circle."

At that moment the thought occurred to me to look at Tom's head. I made him sit down so I could check the mole.

It was gone! Completely Gone!

As an act of praise to God, we went outside with an eight pound hammer, and smashed the fountain to bits. Then we removed it from our land because we wanted everything removed that was connected to that circle.

We cancelled our appointment with the dermatologist and thoroughly celebrated the power of our Risen Christ on Easter Sunday. What a huge blessing this has been.

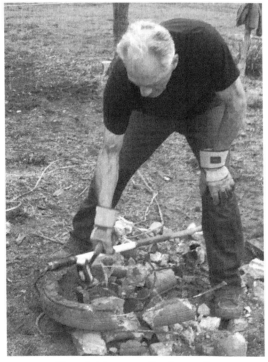

Tom taking out the fountain

On hearing this story, one of the women at church said, "This is really a shock to me because I thought things like this only happened in Africa or California."

No! Supernatural healings happen in Atlanta, Georgia, too!

Healing in an American Restaurant?

Friends of ours, Larry and Anita Parks, are the leaders of ServantCare (www.ServantCare.org), a missionary care ministry providing missionaries on deputation with overnight places to stay (two regional retreat houses as well as a hosted missionary care center in Wisconsin). They also have an effective and extensive prayer chain for missionaries.

(Thanks to both of you for asking your intercessor team to pray for us during our cancer eclipse!)

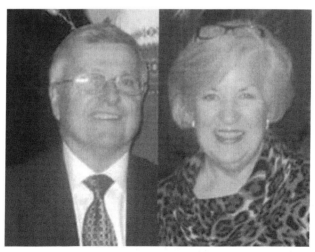

Larry and Anita Parks

The Parks had a wonderful experience of "supernatural touch" healing in a restaurant, of all places. Yes, Jehovah

Rapha is healing Americans in the USA in supernatural touch ways as well as in medical ways!

Here's what they reported:

For dinner we went out to eat with another friend and were waited on by a handsome young man with a bubbly personality who walked with a significant limp. We visited and visited and watched him run around waiting on people with that limp.

After an hour and a half, I turned to Larry and asked, "Do you have faith to pray for him to be healed?" His response was, "I have been sitting here thinking about it."

Ultimately, we called him over to our table, and Larry asked if he believed in God. He said, "Yes." Then Larry asked if he believed God could heal. Again he said, "Yes." Larry asked if he could pray for him and he said, "Yes." So Larry did!

After the prayer, Larry asked the young man to walk for him—he barely had a limp. Big Grin!

We inquired, and he told us he had been in a car accident at six years old which caused a broken pelvis and femur, leaving one leg significantly shorter than the other. Not anymore! They were now the same length!

He also said he had a lot of plastic and metal in his body as a result. So we asked God to replace it with bone. We're hoping that on follow-up visits to the doctor, x-rays will show a miracle had taken place. We are trusting God to do that just as He lengthened his leg. Pray for Brandon.

Curious About the History of Divine / Supernatural Healings?

Here's the record:

1) Supernatural healings are documented in the Old Testament.
2) Supernatural healings by Jesus are documented in the Gospels.
3) Supernatural healings done through the Apostles and New Testament believers are documented in the Book of Acts.
4) Prayers for healing are suggested for believers of all times by James, the brother of Jesus.
5) And, as we see here, supernatural healings are powerfully experienced by many twenty-first century people today!

I, the Lord, do not change!
Malachi. 3:6

Jesus Christ is the same, yesterday, today, and forever!
Hebrews 13:8

APPENDIX D

A Lament Concerning Cancer

By Mark Brewster[72]

Mark and his wife, Jayne, are colleagues of ours who worked with us in Life Impact Ministries. They have a care center in Lewiston, Idaho, which can be found on the Life Impact website. (www.LifeImpactMinistries.net)

Mark had his cancer eclipse diagnosed with a myeloma cancer shortly after I was diagnosed with my cancer. His cancer type was ultimately treated through a stem cell transplant in Seattle. He's also writing a book on his experience, which will be out shortly.

Since cancer is a very discouraging reality, I thought you'd appreciate this "Lament" from Mark, an excerpt from his journal. He certainly captures some of the thoughts I had as well, on my cancer journey.

---

[72] Mark is willing to discuss his situation with anyone interested in learning more. Write him at markkbrewster@gmail.com.

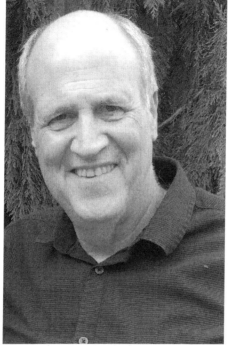

Mark Brewster

Background to My Spewing ...

... I began to realize that cancer was not only a threat to my life, but it was also an inconvenience in my life. It wasn't going away.

So, I wasn't just coming to grips with my own mortality. But this disease had completely disrupted both my personal life and work.

There were endless doctor's appointments and blood draws at the lab. Additionally, I had to go to the cancer center twice a week for infusions during my three months of chemo treatments. So my schedule was filled with having to deal with myeloma.

To this day, I'm extremely grateful that the side effects from the chemo treatments were minimal. However, afterwards I was usually worn out and unable to meet with people or get much of anything done. Though the back pain from the compression fractures was significantly reduced, it was still there and limited my activity.

The stem cell collection and transplant would keep me in Seattle for several months, followed by a lengthy recovery at home and a strong possibility that I would be on maintenance chemo for the rest of my life.

I often jokingly prayed, "Lord, I don't have time to have cancer!" So I was wrestling with both the threat and the inconvenience of my cancer.

I suppose underneath all of this, I was just facing the harsh reality that my battle with myeloma was far from over. By the time I finished my initial chemo treatments I had a touch of battle fatigue. After all, this struggle had been going on for six months.

So, when the doctor told me that I was in remission, my emotions were saying, "At last, we're done with all of this." I knew in my head that wasn't true. But my head wasn't able to convince my feelings of the truth.

Then when we learned that a stem cell transplant would be taking place in just a couple of months and heard about the recovery process and time it would involve, my heart sank. It sank even deeper when we were told about the ongoing procedures and treatments that would be taking place.

It finally hit me that both the threat and inconvenience of my cancer weren't going away. Instead it would always either be immediately in front of me or lurking in the shadows, ready to pounce.

So, one day I decided it was time to lament with the following journal entry. When I write in my journal, I don't worry about grammar, complete sentences, or flow of thought. I just jot down the ramblings of my thoughts and feelings.

You will notice immediately that it's not poetic like a psalm. There's a lot of raw emotion, some of which might even over-exaggerate the circumstances.

Spewing Out My Thoughts ...

It's a lot of spewing out the turmoil in my soul. But there's also the resolve to trust the Lord in spite of it all. I've only edited this in a way to break it down into paragraphs. Here's my psalm...

Spent some time grieving before the Lord that I have cancer. No hostility toward You, Lord — at least that I know of. But I'm sad that I have this illness — at times I feel scared, at times I'm frustrated. But more than anything, I'm in deep grief — and I think that's OK.

Lord, I wish I wasn't sick. I wish I felt good and fully healthy, including my back pain. I wish I could do the things that I used to be able to do — play with my grandkids, take long hikes, go swimming, etc.

I wish I didn't have to wonder if I'll live long enough to see my grandkids grow up, or be in decent enough health to enjoy retirement, if I even make it.

I wish I didn't have to make decisions about what I'm going to do around my chemo schedule, doctor appointments, lab tests, and then, the constantly changing procedures and new appointments that come up.

Lord, I wish this nightmare would end—that I could wake up and everything was better. I wish I could stop wondering if this is the best I'm ever going to feel for the rest of my life. I wish I didn't have to do ministry and life around the uncertainty of how I'm going to feel or what new appointments are going to pop up.

I wish Jayne didn't have to live with the anxiety of where this goes and what it means for her. I wish my kids and grandkids didn't have to live with the fear and concern about my health.

Lord, I'm not asking You to be fair. That's what I deserve, and it would be far worse. I ask that You will be gracious—grant me Your compassionate, healing touch.

Father, you are the giver of every good and perfect gift, in whom there is no variableness or shifting shadow. But quite honestly, I'm having a hard time understanding how this is a good and perfect gift from You. I originally said that it was—but maybe I was just saying that because it sounded right—a way to cope.

Is this a gift from You? Is it? Don't get me wrong—I know You can use it in my life and the lives of others for Your glory. And I embrace that. But my question is: Is this YOUR gift to ME?

Because quite frankly, right now, I can only see it as not just a THREAT to my life...but, also and equally, an inconvenience, a disruption, and limitation—an obstacle—that's in the way of what I believe You called me to DO.

At the same time, this is not a threat, inconvenience, disruption, or an obstacle to what You have called me to BE. I have to admit, that if anything, it has the potential to draw me deeper into Your calling to deeper intimacy with You.

So, in that sense, I can see it as a gift—not so much the illness itself—but Your invitation to me in it. That's the good and perfect gift in this—Your invitation to know You and enjoy You in deeper ways.

But, oh Lord! I desperately need Your grace to embrace and receive this gift. And in embracing and receiving it, I won't relent in asking for Your gift of healing.

In all of this, grant me the grace to say with Jeremiah:

But this I call to mind, and therefore I have hope—
That the steadfast love of Yahweh never ceases.
His mercies (compassions) never come to an end.
They are new every morning,
Great is Your Faithfulness!
The Lord is my portion (everything I need),
says my soul. Therefore I will hope in Him.
— Lamentations 3:22-24

APPENDIX E

Poems & Prayers for Healing

Look Up When Life Causes Us to Look Down!
— Author unknown

The deepest level of worship is …
Praising God in spite of the pain,
Thanking God during the trials,
Trusting Him when we're tempted to lose Hope
and LOVING HIM when He seems
so distant and far away.
At my lowest,
God is my hope.
At my darkest,
God is my light.
At my weakest,
God is my strength.
At my saddest,
God is my comforter.

Is There Any Good in Cancer?
— David Grissen

I personally don't believe there's anything good in cancer, because it's not part of the Kingdom of God, where health reigns. But the results of having cancer can lead to some good in our lives ...

Cancer can be a mover toward repentance
—and who among us doesn't need forgiveness?

Cancer can be a stimulator of faith
—and who among us doesn't need more faith? "Lord, help my unbelief!"

Cancer can be a redeemer of relationships
—and who among us doesn't regret the selfishness we've expressed toward others?

Cancer provides time to consider eternity and one's ultimate destination
—and isn't it prudent to consider the number of our days to gain a heart of wisdom?

So, I guess, those of us fighting cancer or other debilitating diseases could agree with the Apostle Paul:

"And we know that in all things God works for the good of those who love him, who have been called according to his purpose" (Romans 8:31-32).

A Declaration for the Death of Cancer
— David Grissen

O Cancer …
You Thief of Life,
You Mass of Disrupted Cells,
You Cell Essence of Fallen Creation,
You Parasite to the Normal,
You Blaster of Hopes,
You Confounder of Medicine,
You Enemy of Health,
You Absorber of Time's Focus,
You Producer of Pain and Sorrow,
In the Powerful, Mighty, Healing Name of Jesus,
Jehovah Rapha,
We Command You to Shrivel Up and Die!

Praying Promises for Healing
—Anonymous

Heavenly Father,
I thank you for your Living Word. You said that your Word
is life to those who find it and medicine to all their flesh.
Today, by my confession I apply your Word to my body by
giving voice to it.

You said in Psalm 139:14 that I am fearfully and
wonderfully made and that your works are marvelous. I
declare that I am a marvelous creation.

I speak to my body today and declare that I have
authority over it. I command it to receive the Word of God.
Matthew 8:17 proclaims that Jesus bore my sicknesses and
took my infirmities.

Heavenly Father, I thank you that the same Spirit that raised Jesus from the dead dwells in me and makes alive my mortal body.

I speak to my immune system and command it to line up with the Word of God. MY immune system will destroy sickness and disease in my body and perform its job; for this is what God created it to do.

I thank you, Father, that every cell in my body responds to your Word. Your Word permeates my body from the tip of my head to the bottom of my feet. I confess that the Word of God is being made flesh in me.

Psalm 103:3 DECLARES that you, Father, forgave all my iniquities and healed all my diseases. Father, that is your confession, and I make it my confession, also. I don't judge by the sight of my eyes; I judge by your Living Word. It is your Word that lives in me and brings health and healing to every part of my body.

Father, I rejoice at this wonderful promise of spiritual and physical health. Forgive me for my sin, and touch my body with your healing power. Today I ask you to make this promise a reality in my body, soul, and spirit.

Jesus, You paid the price two thousand years ago for spiritual and physical healing. God so loved me that He sent His Son to die on the cross so that I could experience life on God's terms, that is, His abundant life manifesting in me, making me whole—body, soul, and spirit.

In Jesus' Name, AMEN!

APPENDIX F

What Is Your Present Opinion of Jesus?

I've discovered during my seventy-three years of life, both in the USA and abroad, a person can only hold one of four basic opinions about the true identity of Jesus of Nazareth, declared "King of the Jews" by the Roman, Pontius Pilate.

While all four of these views are theoretically possible, I believe it's important to arrive at a decision about which is the most probable based on the evidence.

Otherwise, personal bias of one sort or another could push us to accept a wrong conclusion. Then we would be living on bias—our personal agenda—rather than on solid thinking and accurate decisions.

Here are these four views about Jesus: He's either a LEGEND, a skilled LIAR, a crazy LUNATIC, or a LIVING LORD.

1) The Legend Opinion is that Jesus never really existed historically. Jesus is a fairy tale character, a great story, and an interesting piece of literature, like Jason and the Argonauts.

There is a pile of evidence out there, however, showing Jesus did live on Earth as a historical personality. So it seems this view is more difficult to honestly hold than one of the next three.[73] How do you see it?

2) The Liar Opinion comes from the fact that while Jesus was living his thirty-three years on this earth, He and others made some very outrageous claims about Him. The theory is these claims would be devised so He would have a following as a Jewish Messiah while He lived.

In other words, He said and did things to deceive people into following Him. There have been many religious leaders in history who have gone down this very path!

But Jesus' claims are so outrageous they automatically brand Him and his followers as liars and deceivers...unless, of course, they are true in some way.

For example, here are some of the claims:

---

[73] Mike Mykytuik's has written a number of scholarly articles on historical references for Jesus in *The Bible History Daily* found through this URL:
(https://www.biblicalarchaeology.org/search-results/?cx=008617488963096700126%3As8p_za8hcn0&cof=FORI D%3A10&ie=UTF-8&q=did+Jesus+exist%3F&sa=GO).

- <u>Deity</u>. He claimed to be God and have the power of God, which was demonstrated in certain ways while He was on Earth.[74]

- <u>Resurrection</u>. He also claimed He would die but then within three days come to life again. His stated goal was to destroy the power of death so we could exist with God forever and not rot in the grave.[75] [76]

- <u>Perfection in Humanity</u>. It's claimed about Him that He had no sin, defined as rebellion against God, or falling short in some way of the law God gave us in the ten commandments. In other words, He was a perfect human being.[77]

---

[74] Jesus' statement given to an outcast, a Samaritan woman, in John 4:26, "I who speak to you am He [the Messiah]."

[75] Jesus' statement given in the context of raising a man from the dead in John 11:24, "I am the resurrection and the life. He who believes in me will live, even though he die; and whoever lives and believes in me will never die. Do you believe this?"

[76] "Jesus took the Twelve aside and told them, 'We are going up into Jerusalem, and everything that is written by the prophets about the Son of Man will be fulfilled. He will be handed over to the Gentiles. They will mock him, insult him, spit on him, flog him and kill him. On the third day he will rise again'" (Luke 18:31-33).

[77] "For we do not have a high priest who is unable to sympathize with our weaknesses, but one who in every respect has been tempted as we are, yet without sin" (Hebrews 4:15). This New Testament book deals with the Old Testament priesthood and pictures Jesus as our high priest.

- <u>Truth</u>! He claimed to be truth—that is, the standard for determining what's true and real and what is not. How proud, arrogant, and self-deceiving this claim is if it's not true.[78]

Would you agree these claims are dramatic and self-damning if not true? How easy is it to have someone come out of a coffin in a cemetery and live again after they were buried? I've been to many funerals and never saw this happen.

Would you also agree that IF these claims are not true, it would make Jesus and his disciples BIG liars? He would be a major deceiver and certainly not one I would want to follow!

<u>The Lunatic Opinion</u> would be another view one could hold about Jesus—that He was not really sane. To claim you would die and then come alive again, that you are God, that you have no sin—all these things are claims of someone out of touch with reality. Could His mind have been deranged, or was He a total narcissist?

The only problem with this view is the data we do have about Him in the New Testament Gospels indicates He <u>was not</u> a deranged man.

He was helpful. He was loving to others and treated them well. He spoke common sense to people. He is shown to have supernatural powers which He used in a positive way. He was forgiving. He was gracious. He stood for justice. And He actually healed those

---

[78] "I am the way and the TRUTH and the life. No one comes to the Father except through me" (John 14:6, emphasis mine).

whom society considered lunatics. In fact, He healed many people of various types of sickness and disease.

Outside of this positive picture of Jesus being of the highest character, we simply don't have any data to the contrary. So to consider Him a lunatic is a stretch based on air, not data. Therefore, in my opinion, this view lacks integrity about Jesus. Based on the evidence we have, He was not crazy.

So all of this leaves us with this fact: IF those claims made 2,000 years ago are true, THEN the only wise opinion to have about Jesus of Nazareth, it seems to me, is to agree that He is who He said He was, the Lord of Heaven and Earth.

And if He is Lord, He must be obeyed and given allegiance and reverence by His subjects.

C.S. Lewis, the British atheist-turned-Christian philosopher, speaks to this issue from his experience on both sides of the fence:

> I am trying here to prevent anyone saying the really foolish thing that people often say about Jesus: 'I'm ready to accept Jesus as a great moral teacher, but I don't accept His claim to be God.' That is the one thing we must not say.

> A man who was merely a man and said the sort of things Jesus said would not be a great moral teacher. He would either be a lunatic—on a level with the man who says he is a poached egg—or else he would be the Devil of Hell. You must make your choice.

Either this man was, and is, the Son of God: or else a madman or something worse.[79]

Then Lewis adds:

You can shut Him up for a fool, you can spit at Him and kill Him as a demon; or you can fall at His feet and call Him Lord and God. But let us not come up with any patronizing nonsense about His being a great human teacher. He has not left that open to us. He did not intend to.[80]

Which of the four opinions do you believe is the most probable and why?

---

[79] C. S. Lewis, *Mere Christianity*, London: Collins, 1952, pp. 54-5.

[80] Ibid.

DO YOU WANT TO CONNECT?

Perhaps as you've read my book a question has come to mind you would like answered. Or something I said raised an issue you'd like to discuss further. If so, please let me know. Write me a note with your question or issue, and I'll get back to you.

Write me at: CancerEclipse@gmail.com.
Follow me at: www.GrissenCancerJourney.com

Would You Like Prayer for Your Situation?

If you are fighting cancer and want to be prayed for, please send me a note to that effect, and give us (Sheri and me) your specifics so we can pray with some knowledge about your situation.

Please send this info to: CancerEclipse@gmail.com

- Your name
- Your type of cancer
- Your stage of cancer
- How you're doing in your fight against your cancer

- What you specifically want us to focus on in our intercession for you.

Sheri and I will pray for you that the Lord Jesus Christ, Jehovah Rapha, will bring kingdom healing to your life and into your situation.

We're with you in your battle, as is He!

Write us at: CancerEclipse@gmail.com

How to Order More Books

To order *THE CANCER ECLIPSE: A Path of Hope Forward in Cancer Darkness* go to the website:

www.CancerEclipse.com

(Bulk discounts available. For that, please write me at CancerEclipse@gmail.com)

ABOUT THE AUTHOR

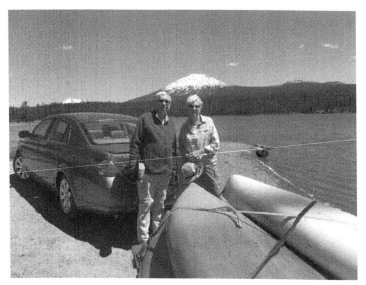

Enjoying life again in Central Oregon, post-cancer battles

Dave Grissen and his wife, Sheri, come from Western Michigan and have been married since September 4, 1968. They have five children and ten grandchildren. Their first great-grandchild is on the way.

Dave and Sheri are both graduates of Hope College in Holland, Michigan. Sheri received a Master's Degree in Christian Counseling from Western Evangelical Seminary in Portland, Oregon. Dave acquired a Masters of Divinity from Western Seminary in Holland, Michigan.

For thirty-two years Dave and Sheri worked internationally for The Navigators, an interdenominational Christian organization, and for Resource Exchange International, a humanitarian aid organization.

First based in Austria for work behind the Iron Curtain, they also had the privilege to live in Germany and Uzbekistan and travel extensively in Europe and beyond.

Dave and Sheri both fought cancer battles and survived. Yes, it is possible!

Made in the USA
San Bernardino, CA
15 February 2018